THE PEDIATRIC HOSPITAL MEDICINE CORE COMPETENCIES

A Framework for Curriculum Development
By the Society of Hospital Medicine

with acknowledgement to pediatric hospitalists from the American Academy of Pediatrics

and

the Academic Pediatric Associat

T0255439

Editors

Erin R. Stucky, MD, FAAP, FHM
University of California San Diego School of Medicine, Department of Pediatrics
Clinical Professor
Vice Chair for Clinical Affairs
Associate Director, Pediatric Residency Program
Fellowship Director, Pediatric Hospital Medicine Program
Rady Children's Hospital San Diego
Director of Graduate Medical Education
Medical Director, Quality Improvement
San Diego, CA

Jennifer Maniscalco, MD, MPH, FAAP
University of Southern California Keck School of Medicine, Department of Pediatrics
Assistant Clinical Professor
Director of Education, Division of Hospital Medicine
Children's Hospital Los Angeles
Los Angeles, CA

Mary C. Ottolini, MD, MPH, FAAP, FHM
George Washington School of Medicine, Department of Pediatrics
Professor of Pediatrics
Vice Chair for Medical Education
Immediate Past Division Chief, Division of Pediatric Hospital Medicine
Children's National Medical Center
Washington, D.C.
Chair, Academic Pediatric Association Education Committee

Statements of Endorsement

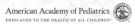

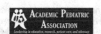

In February 2010, the American Academy of Pediatrics endorsed the following publication: Journal of Hospital Medicine. Pediatric Hospital Medicine Core Competencies (Volume 5: S2) publishing online in April 2010 at www.journalofhospitalmedicine.com.

JOURNAL OF HOSPITAL MEDICINE (ISSN Numbers: Print, 1553-5592; Online, 1553-5606). © 2010 by the Society of Hospital Medicine

The Academic Pediatric Association fully endorses the Pediatric Hospitalist Medicine Core Competencies to define the knowledge skills and attitudes necessary to provide the highest quality of inpatient care for our nation's children. We will continue to lead and collaborate in projects to develop, implement and evaluate educational projects to disseminate the Competencies.

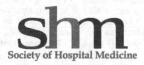

Society of Hospital Medicine

This work was originally published as an online-only supplement to the *Journal of Hospital Medicine* (Volume 5, Supplement 2, 2010). It is available with free and open access online at: www.journalofhospitalmedicine.com.

ISBN: 0 470903589 9780470903582 82304

The *Journal of Hospital Medicine* (Print ISSN 1553-5592; online ISSN 1553-5606 at Wiley InterScience, www.interscience.wiley.com) is published in nine issues per year, one volume per year, for the Society of Hospital Medicine by Wiley Subscription Services, Inc., a Wiley Company, 111 River Street, Hoboken, NJ 07030. Periodicals postage paid at Hoboken, NJ, and at additional mailing offices. Subscription price (Volume 5, 2010): For subscription information, please contact John Wiley & Sons, Inc. (subinfo@wiley.com/201-748-6645). Payment must be made in U.S. dollars drawn on a U.S. bank. Claims for undelivered copies will be accepted only after the following issue has been delivered. Please enclose a copy of the mailing label. Missing copies will be supplied when losses have been sustained in transit and where reserve stock permits. Please allow fourweeks for processing a change of address.

Postmaster: Send address changes to *Journal of Hospital Medicine*, Subscription Distribution, John Wiley & Sons, Inc., 111 River Street, Hoboken, NJ 07030.

Delivery Terms and Legal Title: Prices include delivery of print journals to the recipient's address. Delivery terms are Delivered Duty Unpaid (DDU); the recipient is responsible for paying any import duty or taxes. Legal title passes to the customer on dispatch by our distributors.

Advertising Sales: Inquiries concerning advertising should be directed to: (display advertising) Patrice Culligan, National Account Manager, (212) 904-0369, pculligan@pminy.com; (recruitment) Eamon Wood, Classified Advertising Manager, (212) 904-0363, ewood@pminy.com, Julie Jimenez, Recruitment Advertising Associate (212) 904-0360, jjimenez@pminy.com; Pharmaceutical Media Inc., 30 East 33rd Street, 4th Floor, New York, NY 10016.

Reprints: Reprint sales and inquiries should be directed to the Customer Service Department, John Wiley & Sons, Inc., 111 River Street, Hoboken, NJ 07030. Tel: (201) 748-8789.

Back issues: Single issues from current and recent volumes are available at the current single issue price from cs-journals@wiley.com. Earlier issues may be obtained from Periodicals Service Company, 11 Main Street, Germantown, NY 12526, USA. Tel: +1 518 537 4700, Fax: +1 518 537 5899, Email: psc@periodicals.com.

Other Correspondence: Address all other correspondence to: *Journal of Hospital Medicine*, Publisher, John Wiley & Sons, Inc., 111 River Street, Hoboken, NJ 07030.

For submission instructions, subscription, and all other information visit: http://www.interscience.wiley.com/jhm.

Wiley's Corporate Citizenship initiative seeks to address the environmental, social, economic, and ethical challenges faced in our business and which are important to our diverse stakeholder groups. We have made a long-term commitment to standardize and improve our efforts around the world to reduce our carbon footprint. Follow our progress at www.wiley.com/go/citizenship

∞This paper meets the requirements of ANSI/NISO Z39.48-1992 (Permanence of Paper).

PEDIATRIC HOSPITAL MEDICINE CORE COMPETENCIES

TABLE OF CONTENTS

Section 3:   **SPECIALIZED CLINICAL SERVICES**

Section 4:   **HEALTHCARE SYSTEMS: SUPPORTING AND ADVANCING
CHILD HEALTH**

APPENDIX

Original Research

INTRODUCTION TO THE PEDIATRIC HOSPITAL MEDICINE CORE COMPETENCIES

Background

Pediatric Hospital Medicine continues to evolve as an area of specialization, with the refinement of a distinct knowledgebase and skill set focused on the provision of high quality general pediatric care in the inpatient setting. It is the latest site-specific specialty to emerge from the field of general pediatrics, following a course similar to that charted by pediatric emergency medicine and pediatric critical care medicine in recent decades. The growth of the field has been spurred by a number of factors, including the converging needs for a dedicated emphasis on patient safety, quality improvement, throughput management, and teaching in the inpatient setting.

The number of practicing pediatric hospitalists is estimated to be approximately 2500 and rapidly increasing. To meet the educational needs of this growing cohort of pediatricians, local, regional, and national continuing medical education offerings occur on a regular basis. Furthermore, at least ten fellowships dedicated to advanced training in pediatric hospital medicine have been developed at academic institutions across North America. Despite this, there has been an absence of an accepted and peer-reviewed framework for professional and curriculum development.

The *Pediatric Hospital Medicine Core Competencies* represent the first comprehensive attempt to more formally define the standards for the knowledge, skills, attitudes, and focus on systems improvements that are expected of all pediatric hospitalists, regardless of practice setting or location. It is the culmination of more than five years of planning, research, and development by the Society of Hospital Medicine Pediatric Core Curriculum Task Force, leaders within the Academic Pediatric Association and the American Academy of Pediatrics, and the editorial board. The competencies include contributions from over 80 pediatric hospitalists, content experts, and internal and external reviewers representing university and community hospitals, teaching and non-teaching programs, and key societies and agencies involved in child health from all geographic regions of the United States and Canada. A companion article to *Pediatric Hospital Medicine Core Competencies* in this Supplement provides additional details regarding the project methodology.

Purpose

The *Pediatric Hospital Medicine Core Competencies* provide a framework for professional and curriculum development for all pediatric hospitalists. The framework is intended for use by hospital medicine program directors, directors of medical student clerkships, residency programs, fellowships, and continuing medical education, as well as other educators involved in curriculum development. The competencies do not focus on specific content, but rather general learning objectives within the skills, knowledge, and attitudes related to each topic. Attaining competency in the areas defined in these chapters is expected to require post-residency training. This training is most likely to be obtained through a combination of work experience, local mentorship, and engagement in specific educational programs or fellowship. Pediatric hospitalists, directors, and educators can create specific instructional activities and methods chosen to reflect the characteristics of the intended learners and context of the practice environment.

Organization Structure

The *Pediatric Hospital Medicine Core Competencies* consist of 54 chapters, divided into four sections – Common Clinical Diagnoses and Conditions, Specialized Clinical Services, Core Skills, and Healthcare Systems: Supporting and Advancing Child Health. Within each section, individual chapters on focused topics provide competencies in three domains of educational outcomes: the Cognitive Domain (Knowledge), the Psychomotor Domain (Skills), and the Affective Domain (Attitudes). To reflect the emphasis of hospital medicine practice on improving healthcare systems, a fourth section entitled Systems Organization and Improvement is also included. An attempt has been made to make the objectives "timeless", allowing for creation of curriculum that can be nimble and reactive to new discoveries. Highly specific temporal changes in medicine are purposefully excluded, and instead the focus is on the drivers for these changes or advancements. Phrases and wording were selected to help guide the learning activities most likely to achieve each competency and to reflect the varied roles that pediatric hospitalists have in different practice settings. In this document, the terms "child" and "children" include infants, children, adolescents, and young adults up to the age of 21, in accordance of policies of the American Academy of Pediatrics. However, it is also understood that care is rendered in pediatric settings for patients who may surpass this upper age limit based on diagnosis or special healthcare needs. Finally, although the entire document can be a resource for comprehensive program development, each chapter is intended to stand alone and thus support curriculum development specific to the needs of individual programs.

Conclusion and Acknowledgement

The *Pediatric Hospital Medicine Core Competencies* are intended to provide standards for the knowledge, skills, and attitudes expected of all pediatric hospitalists and to provide a framework for ongoing professional and curriculum development for learners at all levels. We welcome feedback and evaluation from pediatric hospitalists and from all with whom we partner to improve the care for hospitalized children.

We wish to acknowledge the dedication of authors and associate editors, and the thoughtful review by the members of hospital organizations, accrediting bodies, and agencies listed in this supplement. This inaugural edition of the *Pediatric Hospital Medicine Core Competencies* should serve as the foundation from which the field of Pediatric Hospital Medicine will continue to evolve. We look forward with anticipation to future revisions as we reflect on our goals and advance our field.

The *Pediatric Hospital Medicine Core Competencies* Editorial Board

Erin Stucky, MD
Mary C Ottolini, MD, MPH
Jennifer Maniscalco, MD, MPH

AUTHORS

Rishi Agrawal, MD, MPH
Pediatric Hospitalist, Children's Memorial Hospital and LaRabida Children's Hospital
Assistant Professor of Pediatrics, Northwestern University Feinberg School of Medicine
Chicago, IL
Feeding Tubes

Brian Alverson, MD
Head, Pediatric Hospitalist Section, Hasbro Children's Hospital
Assistant Professor of Pediatrics, Warren Alpert School of Medicine at Brown University
Providence, RI
Neonatal Fever
Pneumonia

Allison Ballantine, MD
Medical Director of the Integrated Care Service, Children's Hospital of Philadelphia
Assistant Professor of Pediatrics, University of Pennsylvania School of Medicine
Philadelphia, PA
Technology Dependent Children

Julia Beauchamp-Walters, MD
Pediatric Emergency Transport Coordinator, CSSD, RCHHC Pediatric Emergency Transports,
Rady Childrens Hospital
Clinical Instructor of Pediatrics, University of California, San Diego
San Diego, CA
Transport of the Critically Ill Child

Glenn F. Billman, MD
Medical Safety and Regulatory Officer, Rady Children's Hospital
San Diego, CA
Patient Safety

April O. Buchanan, MD, FAAP
Vice Chair of Quality, Department of Pediatrics, Children's Hospital at Greenville Hospital
System University Medical Center
Assistant Professor of Clinical Pediatrics, University of South Carolina School of Medicine
Greenville, SC
Shock

Douglas W. Carlson, MD
Chief, Pediatric Hospital Medicine, St. Louis Children's Hospital
Associate Professor of Pediatrics, Washington University
St. Louis, MO
Procedural Sedation
Technology Dependent Children

Vincent W. Chiang, MD
Chief, Inpatient Services, Department of Medicine, Children's Hospital Boston
Associate Professor of Pediatrics, Harvard Medical School
Boston, MA
Seizures

Michael R. Clemmens, MD
Director Pediatric Hospitalist Program, Anne Arundel Medical Center
Assistant Clinical Professor of Pediatrics, The George Washington University School of Medicine
Annapolis, MD
Acute Abdominal Pain and The Acute Abdomen

Jamie L. Clute, MD, FAAP, FHM
Medical Director, Inpatient Services, Joe Dimaggio Children's Hospital
Clinical Assistant Professor, NOVA Southeastern University, College of Osteopathic Medicine and
Assistant Affiliate Professor, Barry University
Hollywood, FL
Kawasaki Disease

Shannon Connor Phillips, MD, MPH
Patient Safety Officer, Quality and Patient Safety Institute, Cleveland Clinic
Assistant Professor of Pediatrics, Cleveland Clinic Lerner College of Medicine at
Case Western Reserve University
Cleveland, OH
Evidence Based Medicine

Tanya Dansky, MD
Medical Director, Children's Physicians Medical GroupMedical Director, San Diego Hospice and The Institute
For Palliative Medicine, Rady Children's Hospital
Assistant Clinical Professor of Pediatrics, University of California, San Diego
San Diego, CA
Hospice and Palliative Care, Ethics

Jennifer Daru, MD, FAAP, FHM
Chief, Pediatric Hospitalist Division; Interim Chief, Pediatric and Neonatal Transport, California Pacific
Medical Center
Clinical Assistant Professor (pending), University of California San Francisco
San Francisco, CA
Leading a Healthcare Team
Newborn Care and Delivery Room Management

Yasmeen N. Daud, MD
Director of Pediatric Hospitalist Sedation in the Pediatric Acute Wound Service and Director of the Pediatric
Hospitalist After Hours Sedation Program, St. Louis Children's Hospital
Assistant Professor of Pediatrics, Washington University School of Medicine
St. Louis, MO
Oxygen Delivery and Airway Management

Craig DeWolfe, MD, MEd
Pediatric Hospitalist, Children's National Medical Center
Assistant Professor of Pediatrics, George Washington School of Medicine and Health Sciences
Washington DC
Apparent Life-Threatening Event

Joseph M. Geskey, DO
Division Chief, Pediatric Hospital Medicine, Medical Director of Hospital Care Management,
Penn State Hershey Children's Hospital
Associate Professor of Pediatrics, Penn State M. S. Hershey Medical Center
Hershey, PA
Pneumonia
Upper Airway Infections
Bronchiolitis

Paul D. Hain, MD
Associate Chief of Staff, Monroe Carell Jr. Children's Hospital at Vanderbilt
Assistant Professor of Pediatrics, Vanderbilt University
Nashville, TN
Health Information Systems

Keith Herzog, MD
Pediatric Hospitalist, St. Christopher's Hospital for Children
Assistant Professor of Pediatrics, Drexel University College of Medicine
Philadelphia, PA
Central Nervous System Infections

Margaret Hood, MD, FAAP
Pediatric Hospitalist, Seattle Children's Hospital
Clinical Associate Professor of Pediatrics, University of Washington
Seattle, WA
Diabetes Mellitus
Hospice and Palliative Care

Kevin B. Johnson, MD, MS
Vice Chair of Biomedical Informatics, Vanderbilt University Medical Center
Associate Professor of Medical Informatics and Pediatrics, Vanderbilt University Medical Center
Nashville, TN
Health Information Systems

Rick Johnson, MD, FAAP
> Division Head, Regional Pediatrics, CCMC, and American Heart Association Regional and National PALS
> Faculty, Connecticut Children's Medical Center
> Assistant Professor of Pediatrics, University of Connecticut School of Medicine
> Hartford, CT
> *Pediatric Advanced Life Support*

Brian Kelly, MD, MRCP (UK), FAAP
> Pediatric Hospitalist, Ranken Jordan Pediatric Rehabilitative Hospital, St. Louis Children's Hospital
> Assistant Professor of Pediatrics, Washington University School of Medicine
> St. Louis, MO
> *Bladder Catheterization/Suprapubic Bladder Tap*

Herbert C Kimmons, MD, MMM
> President Children's Specialists of San Diego (Medical Quality Officer of Rady Children's Hospital of
> San Diego, 2006-2008), Children's Specialists of San Diego in California
> Professor of Pediatrics, University of California San Diego
> San Diego, CA
> *Continuous Quality Improvement*
> *Patient Safety*

Su-Ting T. Li, MD, MPH
> Associate Pediatric Residency Program Director, University of California, Davis
> Assistant Professor of Pediatrics, University of California, Davis
> Sacramento, CA
> *Skin and Soft Tissue Infections*

Patricia S. Lye, MD
> Medical Director, Hospitalists, Children's Hospital of Wisconsin
> Associate Professor of Pediatrics, Medical College of Wisconsin
> Milwaukee, WI
> *Transitions of Care*

Jennifer Maniscalco, MD, MPH, FAAP
> Director of Education, Division of Pediatric Hospital Medicine, Children's Hospital Los Angeles
> Clinical Assistant Professor of Pediatrics, University of Southern California Keck School of Medicine
> Los Angeles, CA
> *Failure to Thrive*
> *Transitions of Care*
> *Nutrition*

David E. Marcello III, MD, FAAP
> Pediatric Hospitalist, Connecticut Children's Medical Center
> Assistant Professor in Pediatrics, University of Connecticut Medical School
> Hartford, CT
> *Lumbar Puncture*
> *Intravenous Access and Phlebotomy*

Sanford M. Melzer, MD, MBA
> Senior Vice President, Strategic Planning and Business Development, Seattle Children's Hospital
> Professor of Pediatrics, University of Washington School of Medicine
> Seattle, WA
> *Cost Effective Care*

Margaret I. Mikula, MD
> Pediatric Hospitalist, Penn State Hershey Children's Hospital
> Assistant Professor of Pediatrics, Penn State M. S. Hershey Medical Center
> Hershey, PA
> *Pneumonia*
> *Bronchiolitis*

Laura J Mirkinson, MD, FAAP
> Director of Pediatrics, Blythedale Children's Hospital
> Valhalla, NY
> *Neonatal Jaundice*

Christopher D. Miller, MD, FAAP
Pediatric Hospitalist and Allergist, Children's Mercy Hospitals and Clinics
Assistant Professor of Pediatrics, University of Missouri-Kansas City School of Medicine
Kansas City, MO
Asthma

Christopher O'Hara, MD, FACP
St. Christopher's Hospital for Children
Assistant Professor of Pediatrics, Drexel University College of Medicine
Philadelphia PA
Pain Management

Mary C. Ottolini MD, MPH, FAAP, FHM
Chair, Academic Pediatric Association Education Committee
Immediate Past Hospitalist Division Chief; Vice Chair for Medical Education, Children's National Medical Center
Professor of Pediatrics, The George Washington University School of Medicine
Washington DC
Fluid and Electrolyte Management
Gastroenteritis
Education

Brian M. Pate, MD, FAAP, FHM
Section Chief, Pediatric Hospital Medicine, Vice Chairman, Inpatient Services, Children's Mercy Hospital and Clinics
Assistant Professor of Pediatrics, University of Missouri-Kansas City School of Medicine
Business Practices
Asthma

Dana Patrick, RN, BSN
Transport Program Manager NICU\PICU, Rady Children's Hospital
San Diego, CA
Transport of the Critically Ill Child

Jack M. Percelay, MD, MPH, FAAP, FHM
Society of Hospital Medicine, Pediatric Board Member; Immediate Past-Chair, AAP Section on
Hospital Medicine, E.L.M.O. Pediatrics
Associate Professor, Pace University Physician Assistant Program
New York, New York
Advocacy

David Pressel, MD, PhD, FHM, FAAP
Director, General Pediatrics Inpatient Services, A.I. duPont Hospital for Children
Assistant Professor of Pediatrics, Jefferson Medical College, Thomas Jefferson University
Wilmington, DE
Child Abuse and Neglect

Kris P Rehm, MD
Director, Division of Hospital Medicine, Monroe Carell Jr Children's Hospital at Vanderbilt
Assistant Professor of Pediatrics, Vanderbilt University
Nashville, TN
Respiratory Failure

Kyung E. Rhee, MD, MSc
Pediatric Hospitalist, Hasbro Children's Hospital and The Weight Control and Diabetes Research Center
Assistant Professor of Pediatrics, Warren Alpert Medical School of Brown University
Providence, RI
Fever of Unknown Origin

Mark F Riederer, MD
Pediatric Hospitalist, Monroe Carell Jr Children's Hospital at Vanderbilt
Assistant Professor of Pediatrics,
Nashville, TN
Respiratory Failure

Michael Ruhlen, MD, MHCM, FAAP, FHM, FACHE
Vice President and Chief Medical Officer, Carolinas Medical Center – Mercy
Carolinas Medical Center – Pineville
Charlotte, NC
Legal Issues/Risk Management

Henry M. Seidel, MD
    Professor Emeritus, Johns Hopkins Berman Institute of Bioethics
    Professor Emeritus of Pediatrics, The Johns Hopkins University School of Medicine
    Baltimore, MD
    Communication

Anand Sekaran, MD
    Medical Director, Inpatient Services, Connecticut Children's Medical Center
    Assistant Professor of Pediatrics, University of Connecticut School of Medicine
    Hartford, CT
    Radiographic Interpretation

Kristin A. Shadman, MD, FAAP
    Pediatric Hospitalist
    Oxygen Delivery and Airway Management

Vipul Singla, MD, FAAP
    Site Leader, Lake Forest Hospital (Children's Memorial Medical Group)
    Instructor in Pediatrics, Northwestern University Feinberg School of Medicine
    Chicago, IL
    Electrocardiogram Interpretation

Karen Smith, MD, MEd
    Chief Medical Officer, The HSC Pediatric Center
    Assistant Professor of Pediatrics, The George Washington University School of Medicine
    Washington DC
    Apparent Life-Threatening Event

Jeffrey L. Sperring, MD
    Chief Medical Officer, Riley Hospital for Children
    Assistant Professor of Pediatrics, Indiana University School of Medicine
    Indianapolis, IN
    Bone and Joint Infections

Glenn Stryjewski, MD, MPH
    Associate Residency Program Director, AI duPont Hospital for Children
    Assistant professor of Pediatrics, Jefferson Medical College, Thomas Jefferson University
    Wilmington, DE
    Toxic Ingestion

Erin R. Stucky, MD, FAAP, FHM
    Director of Graduate Medical Education, Rady Children's Hospital San Diego; Medical Director of Quality
    Improvement, Rady Children's Hospital San Diego; Associate Program Director, UCSD Pediatric Residency Program;
    Vice Chair for Clinical Affairs, UCSD Department of Pediatrics; Director, Pediatric Hospital Medicine Fellowship,
    Rady Children's Hospital
    Clinical Professor of Pediatrics, University of California San Diego
    San Diego, CA
    Evidence Based Medicine
    Continuous Quality Improvement
    Technology Dependent Children

E. Douglas Thompson, Jr., MD
    Director, Pediatric Generalist Service, St. Christopher's Hospital for Children
    Assistant Professor of Pediatrics, Drexel University College of Medicine
    Philadelphia, PA
    Sickle Cell Disease

Michael Turmelle, MD
    Pediatric Hospitalist, St. Louis Children's Hospital
    Assistant Professor of Pediatrics, Washington University School of Medicine
    St. Louis, MO
    Non-Invasive Monitoring

Macdara G. Tynan, MD, MBA, FAAP
Associate Director of Inpatient Pediatrics, Levine Children's Hospital
Charlotte, NC
Diabetes Mellitus
Toxic Ingestion

Ronald J. Williams, MD
Pediatric Hospitalist, Penn State Hershey Children's Hospital
Associate Professor of Pediatrics and Medicine, Penn State M. S. Hershey Medical Center
Hershey, PA
Upper Airway Infections

Heidi Wolf MD, FAAP
Director Pediatric Hospitalist Program, Johns Hopkins
Assistant Clinical Professor, John Hopkins University
Baltimore, MD
Fever of Unknown Origin
Neonatal Fever

Susan Wu, MD
Pediatric Hospitalist, Children's Hospital Los Angeles
Clinical Assistant Professor of Pediatrics, University of Southern California Keck School of Medicine
Los Angeles, CA
Bronchiolitis

Lisa B. Zaoutis, MD
Section Chief of Inpatient Services, Division of General Pediatrics, The Children's Hospital of Philadelphia
Assistant Professor of Pediatrics, University of Pennsylvania School of Medicine
Philadelphia, PA
Urinary Tract Infections

William T. Zempsky, MD
Associate Director; Division of Pain Medicine; Department of Pediatrics, Associate Director,
Pain Relief Program, Connecticut Children's Medical Center
Professor of Pediatrics, University of Connecticut School of Medicine
Hartford, CT
Pain Management

REVIEWERS

Allison Ballantine, MD
Medical Director of the Integrated Care Service, Children's Hospital of Philadelphia
Assistant Professor of Pediatrics, University of Pennsylvania School of Medicine
Philadelphia, PA
Technology Dependent Children

Margaret Hood, MD, FAAP
Pediatric Hospitalist, Seattle Children's Hospital
Clinical Associate Professor of Pediatrics, University of Washington
Seattle, WA
Hospice and Palliative Care
Ethics

Brian Kit, MD, MPH
Anne Arundel Medical Center
Assistant Professor of Pediatrics, The George Washington University School of Medicine
Annapolis, MD
Advocacy

Evelina M. Krieger, MD
Children's National Medical Center
Assistant Professor of Pediatrics, The George Washington University School of Medicine
Washington, DC
Advocacy

Cynthia L. Kuelbs, MD
>Medical Director, Chadwick Center for Child Abuse; Division Director Pediatric Hospital Medicine,
>Rady Children's Hospital
>Associate Clinical Professor of Pediatrics, University of California San Diego
>San Diego, CA
>*Child Abuse and Neglect*

Christopher P. Landrigan, MD, MPH
>Division Director, Pediatrics and Hospital Medicine; Research and Fellowship Director,
>Children's Hospital Boston Inpatient Pediatrics Service; Director,
>Sleep and Patient Safety Program at the Brigham and Women's Hospital,
>Children's Hospital Boston
>Assistant Professor of Pediatrics and Medicine, Harvard Medical School
>Boston, MA
>*Research*

Michael Ruhlen, MD, MHCM, FAAP, FHM, FACHE
>Vice President and Chief Medical Officer, Carolinas Medical Center – Mercy
>Carolinas Medical Center – Pineville
>Charlotte, NC
>*Legal Issues/Risk Management*

Samir S. Shah, MD, MSCE
>Senior Scholar, Center for Clinical Epidemiology and Biostatistics, The Children's Hospital of Philadelphia
>Assistant Professor, Departments of Pediatrics and Biostatistics and Epidemiology, University of Pennsylvania
>School of Medicine
>Philadelphia, PA
>*Research*

Rajendu Srivastava, MD, FRCP(C), MPH
>Director of Pediatric Research in the Inpatient Setting (PRIS) Network,
>Primary Children's Medical Center, Intermountain Healthcare Inc.
>Associate Professor, Division of Inpatient Medicine, Department of Pediatrics,
>University of Utah Health Sciences Center
>Salt Lake City, UT
>*Research*

Ben Bauer, MD, FAAP
>Pediatric Hospital Medicine; Fellowship Director, Riley Children's Hospital, Indiana University School of Medicine
>Indianapolis, IN

John Combes, MD
>President/COO, Center for Healthcare Governance, American Hospital Association (AHA)
>Washington, DC

Jennifer Daru, MD, FAAP, FHM
>Chair-elect AAP; Section on Hospital Medicine, American Academy of Pediatrics
>San Francisco, CA

Jerrold Eichner, MD, FAAP
>Chair, AAP National Committee on Hospital Care, American Academy of Pediatrics
>Great Falls, MT

Rosemarie Faber, MSN/ED, RN, CCRN
>Clinical Practice Specialist, American Association of Critical Care Nurses
>Aliso Viejo, CA

Rani S Gereige, MD, MPH, FAAP
>Director of Medical Education, Miami Children's Hospital
>Miami, FL

David Jaimovich, MD, FAAP
>President, QRI (Former Chief Medical Officer and Vice President for International Accreditation Services for
>Joint Commission Resources (JCR) and Joint Commission International (JCI)), Quality Resources International

Andrea Kline RN, MS, CPNP-AC, CCRN, FCCM
>Executive Board; Professional Issues; Pediatric Critical Care NP, National Association of Pediatric Nurse
>Practitioners (NAPNAP)
>Cherry Hill, NJ

David D. Lloyd, MD, FRCP(C), FAAP
Section Chief of General Pediatrics Children's Healthcare of Atlanta,
Director of Undergraduate Pediatric Education, Director of the Pediatric Hospitalist Fellowship,
Children's Healthcare of Atlanta, Emory University School of Medicine
Atlanta, GA

Patricia S. Lye, MD, FAAP
AAP Section on Hospital Medicine, American Academy of Pediatrics
Milwaukee, WI

Sanjay Mahant, MD, FRCPC
Pediatric Hospital Medicine Fellowship Director, Hospital for Sick Children,
University of Toronto School of Medicine
Toronto, Canada

Jennifer Maniscalco, MD, MPH, FAAP
Pediatric Hospital Medicine Fellowship Director, Children's Hospital Los Angeles
University of Southern California School of Medicine

Marlene Miller, MD, MSc, FAAP
Vice President for Quality, National Association of Children's Hospitals and Related Institutions (NACHRI)
Alexandria, VA

Paul E. Manicone, MD, FAAP
Associate Division Chief; Division of Hospitalist Medicine; Immediate past Fellowship Director,
Children's National Medical Center, George Washington University School of Medicine
Washington DC

Warren Newton, MD
American Board of Family Medicine Board of Directors: Research and Development, IT, and
Communications/publications Committees; Executive Associate Dean for Medical Education and
William B. Aycock Distinguished Professor and Chair, Department of Family Medicine at the University of
North Carolina at Chapel Hill, American Board of Family Medicine
Lexington, KY

Daniel Rauch, MD, FAAP, FHM
Chair, AAP Section on Hospital Medicine; Immediate Past Chair, Academic Pediatric Association
Hospital Medicine Special Interest Group
AAP and APA

Ellen Schwalenstocker, PhD, MBA
Quality, Advocacy and Measurement, NACHRI
Alexandria, VA

Mary Jean Schuman, MSN, MBA, RN, CPNP
Chief Programs Officer, American Nursing Association
Silver Spring, MD

Neha H. Shah, MD, FAAP
Fellowship Director, Pediatric Hospital Medicine, Children's National Medical Center
George Washington University School of Medicine
Washington, DC

Geeta Singhal, MD, FAAP
Director, Pediatric Hospital Medicine Fellowship; Director, Faculty Inpatient Service; Co-Director,
PEM Faculty Development Program, Texas Children's Hospital, Baylor College of Medicine
Houston, TX

Jeffrey L. Sperring, MD, FAAP
Chair, Academic Pediatric Association Hospital Medicine Special Interest Group
Chief Medical Officer, Academic Pediatric Association
Indianapolis, IN

Erin R. Stucky, MD, FAAP, FHM
Pediatric Hospital Medicine, Fellowship Director, Rady Children's Hospital San Diego
University of California San Diego School of Medicine
San Diego, CA

EDITORS

Michael G. Burke, MD, MBA
 Chairman of Pediatrics, Saint Agnes Hospital
 Assistant Professor of Pediatrics, The Johns Hopkins University School of Medicine
 Baltimore, MD

Douglas W. Carlson, MD
 Chief, Pediatric Hospital Medicine, St. Louis Children's Hospital
 Associate Professor of Pediatrics, Washington University
 St. Louis, MO

Timothy T. Cornell, MD
 C. S. Mott Women and Children's Hospital
 Assistant Professor in the Department of Pediatrics and Communicable Diseases, University of Michigan
 Ann Arbor, MI

Jack M. Percelay, MD, MPH, FAAP, FHM
 Society of Hospital Medicine, Pediatric Board Member; Immediate Past-Chair, AAP Section on Hospital
 Medicine, E.L.M.O. Pediatrics
 Associate Professor, Pace University Physician Assistant Program
 New York, New York

Daniel Rauch, MD, FAAP, FHM
 Associate Director of Pediatrics, Elmhurst Hospital
 New York

Anand Sekaran, MD
 Medical Director, Inpatient Services, Connecticut Children's Medical Center
 Assistant Professor of Pediatrics, University of Connecticut School of Medicine
 Hartford, CT

E. Douglas Thompson, Jr., MD
 Director, Pediatric Generalist Service, St. Christopher's Hospital for Children
 Assistant Professor of Pediatrics, Drexel University College of Medicine
 Philadelphia, PA

Heidi Wolf MD, FAAP
 Director Pediatric Hospitalist Program, Johns Hopkins
 Assistant Clinical Professor, John Hopkins University
 Baltimore, MD

David Zipes, MD FAAP, FHM
 Director, St. Vincent Pediatric Hospitalists, Peyton Manning Children's Hospital at St. Vincent
 Indianapolis, IN

SENIOR EDITORS

Jennifer Maniscalco, MD, MPH, FAAP
 Director of Education, Division of Pediatric Hospital Medicine, Children's Hospital Los Angeles
 Clinical Assistant Professor of Pediatrics, University of Southern California Keck School of Medicine
 Los Angeles, CA

Mary C. Ottolini MD, MPH, FAAP, FHM
 Chair, Academic Pediatric Association Education Committee
 Immediate Past Hospitalist Division Chief; Vice Chair for Medical Education, Children's National Medical Center
 Professor of Pediatrics, The George Washington University School of Medicine
 Washington DC

Erin R. Stucky, MD, FAAP, FHM
 Director of Graduate Medical Education, Rady Children's Hospital San Diego;
 Medical Director of Quality Improvement, Rady Children's Hospital San Diego;
 Associate Program Director, UCSD Pediatric Residency Program;
 Vice Chair for Clinical Affairs, UCSD Department of Pediatrics;
 Director, Pediatric Hospital Medicine Fellowship, Rady Children's Hospital
 Clinical Professor of Pediatrics, University of California San Diego
 San Diego, CA

Pediatric Hospital Medicine Core Competencies

Section One: Common Clinical Diagnoses and Conditions

ACUTE ABDOMINAL PAIN AND THE ACUTE ABDOMEN

INTRODUCTION

Acute abdominal pain is a common presenting symptom of children and adolescents and prompts the consideration of an extensive differential diagnosis. Although it is frequently due to common, self-limited medical conditions related to the abdomen such as gastroenteritis, it may also be a signal of systemic illness or referred from problems elsewhere in the body. Acute abdominal pain may or may not be accompanied by signs and symptoms of an acute abdomen such as loss of bowel sounds or evidence of obstruction. Identifying children with a true medical or surgical emergency is critical. Children with peritonitis and other surgical conditions need prompt evaluation by a surgeon with pediatric expertise. Early diagnosis and treatment reduces morbidity, mortality, and length of hospital stay. Pediatric hospitalists frequently encounter children with acute abdominal pain in a variety of clinical settings and should assist in the timely and effective evaluation and management either alone or in conjunction with a surgeon.

KNOWLEDGE

Pediatric hospitalists should be able to:

- Recognize features of the medical history and physical examination that prompt specific diagnostic evaluation.
- Describe the differential diagnosis of acute abdominal pain as well the acute abdomen for children of varying chronological and developmental ages.
- List gender-specific etiologies of acute abdominal pain, such as testicular torsion and ovarian cyst rupture.
- Identify the role congenital anomalies may play in the child with an acute abdomen.
- Discuss the principles of stabilization of the child with an acute abdomen, such as volume resuscitation, antibiotics, and bowel decompression.
- List conditions that may mimic the acute abdomen, such as lower lobe pneumonia and diabetic ketoacidosis.
- State the importance of, and indications for, early surgical consultation in the child with an acute abdomen.
- Compare and contrast benefits versus limitations of various commonly performed studies such as acute abdominal series, sonography, computed tomography, nuclear medicine scans, and magnetic resonance imaging. State the benefits of and barriers to use of contrast enhancement for these studies.
- Provide indications for hospital admission and cite the reasons for admission to various locations in the hospital system, such as a short-stay unit, surgical or medical ward, step-down intensive care unit, or intensive care unit.
- Cite reasons for patient transfer to a referral center in cases requiring pediatric-specific services not available at the local facility.
- Identify specific evaluation and treatment needs for technology dependent children who present with an acute abdomen, including children with feeding and drainage tubes (gastrostomy, jejunostomy, ileosotomy, and others), long term vascular access devices (ports, Hickman catheters, and others), shunts (ventricular, other), ventilator dependence, and other implanted devices.
- Summarize the approach toward pain control in patients presenting with acute abdominal pain, attending to medication choice, delivery method, and impact on exam re-assessments.

SKILLS

Pediatric hospitalists should be able to:

- Obtain an accurate history and perform a thorough physical examination.
- Formulate a targeted differential diagnosis based on elements from the history and physical examination, prior to ordering studies.
- Identify the child with an acute abdomen.
- Identify and manage the child with concomitant hypovolemia or sepsis.
- Direct an appropriate and cost-effective evaluation to identify the cause of the abdominal pain or the acute abdomen.
- Access radiology services efficiently, for both performance and interpretation of studies.
- Order and correctly interpret commonly performed basic diagnostic imaging studies and laboratory studies.
- Consult surgeons effectively and efficiently when indicated.
- Identify the child requiring emergent surgical consultation.

- Provide pre- and post-operative general pediatric care for the child requiring surgery, as appropriate, including pain management.
- Coordinate care with the primary care provider and arrange an appropriate transition plan for hospital discharge.

ATTITUDES

Pediatric hospitalists should be able to:
- Assume responsibility for care of patients as the primary attending or in collaboration with the surgical team.
- Communicate effectively with patients, the family/caregiver, and healthcare providers regarding findings and care plans.

SYSTEMS ORGANIZATION AND IMPROVEMENT

In order to improve efficiency and quality within their organizations, pediatric hospitalists should:
- Educate healthcare providers, trainees, the family/caregiver regarding the signs and symptoms of the acute abdomen to encourage early detection and prompt evaluation.
- Lead, coordinate or participate in a multidisciplinary team to provide optimal care for children with acute abdominal pain with and without acute abdomen.
- Incorporate knowledge of outcomes research and cost management strategies into the evaluation and treatment of patients with an acute abdomen.
- Lead, coordinate or participate in institutional efforts to improve the expediency of diagnostic laboratory and radiographic studies, availability of specialty care, and other resources for patients with acute abdominal pain and acute abdomen.

APPARENT LIFE-THREATENING EVENT

INTRODUCTION

Apparent Life-Threatening Event (ALTE) is defined by the NIH Consensus Development Conference on Infantile Apnea and Home Monitoring as an episode that is frightening to the observer and that is characterized by some combination of apnea (central or occasionally obstructive), color change (usually cyanotic or pallid but occasionally erythematous or plethoric), marked change in muscle tone (usually marked limpness), choking, or gagging. Because ALTE is a description of symptoms rather than a diagnosis, epidemiologic data is imprecise. It is estimated that 1-3% of infants will have an episode that can be described as an ALTE and that most of these infants present before 2 months of life. Pediatric hospitalists can provide a valuable service to the family/caregiver by reconciling the potentially life threatening nature of ALTE with an infant who often appears normal on physical examination. Pediatric hospitalists should approach the broad differential diagnosis in a logical, systematic manner.

KNOWLEDGE

Pediatric hospitalists should be able to:
- Describe the differential diagnosis of ALTE (such as gastroesophageal reflux disease, seizure, apnea of prematurity, infection [sepsis, meningitis, pertussis, bronchiolitis], toxin, breath-holding spell, cardiac arrhythmia, obstructive sleep apnea, inborn errors of metabolism, central hypoventilation syndrome, hydrocephalus, child abuse, Munchausen's Syndrome by Proxy, and others) and the key historical or physical findings specifically associated with each diagnosis.
- Provide indications for admission to the hospital and determine the appropriate level of care required.
- Describe the goals of hospitalization including stabilization, diagnosis, treatment, reassurance, and education.
- Compare and contrast Sudden Infant Death Syndrome (SIDS) versus ALTE,
- Discuss current hypotheses regarding the etiology of SIDS and relate this to the spectrum of disorders that may cause ALTE.
- Describe a basic approach toward the work-up for ALTE and list the factors that may warrant an increased level of laboratory, radiographic, or other testing.
- Summarize the literature on the impact of home monitors on morbidity and mortality and identify the benefits and limitations of home monitoring.

SKILLS

Pediatric hospitalists should be able to:
- Resuscitate and stabilize an infant with ALTE who presents in an unstable state.
- Obtain an accurate patient history and perform a thorough physical examination eliciting features to narrow the differential diagnosis of ALTE.
- Critically assess the level of evidence and risk/benefit ratio for the diagnostic work-up and management plan.
- Interpret basic tests (such as laboratory tests, chest x-rays, and electrocardiograms) and identify abnormal findings that require further testing or consultation.
- Order appropriate monitoring and correctly interpret monitor data.
- Engage consultants and support staff (such as subspecialty physicians and social workers) efficiently and appropriately.
- Use the ALTE admission as an opportunity to educate the family/caregiver on proper sleep positioning and risk factors for SIDS.
- Impart basic resuscitation skills to the family/caregiver, using a teach-back method.
- Coordinate care with the primary care provider and arrange an appropriate transition plan for hospital discharge.

ATTITUDES

Pediatric hospitalists should be able to:
- Communicate effectively with the family/caregiver, and healthcare providers regarding findings and care plans.
- Ensure a safe and supportive atmosphere for the patient and family during the period of observation and evaluation of a child admitted following an ALTE.
- Counsel the family/caregiver on the valid use of home monitors in a limited population, noting the features which support or refute use of a home monitor for their child.
- Realize the impact of an ALTE on the family/caregiver and the implications for discharge planning and follow-up.
- Role model professional behavior when addressing issues related to potential social concerns and child abuse evaluation.

SYSTEMS ORGANIZATION AND IMPROVEMENT

In order to improve efficiency and quality within their organizations, pediatric hospitalists should:
- Lead, coordinate or participate in multidisciplinary initiatives to develop and implement evidence-based clinical guidelines to improve quality of care for infants with ALTE.
- Advocate for preventive education regarding sudden infant death syndrome in the hospital system and community.

ASTHMA

INTRODUCTION

Asthma is the most common childhood chronic disease and is the third leading cause of hospital admission for children less than 15 years of age. Prevalence and mortality rates have increased over the past decade, along with costs, the latter predominantly associated with hospital based care. The Department of Health and Human Services (DHHS), through the National Institutes of Health (NIH), coordinated the National Asthma Education and Prevention Program designed to provide up-to-date evidence-based guidelines for the diagnosis, treatment and prevention of asthma. The DHHS also identified asthma as one of the key elements of the Healthy People 2010 initiative with several specific health objectives related directly to inpatient management. Due to the chronic nature of this disease, pediatric hospitalists should not only treat the acute exacerbation resulting in status asthmaticus, but also create or re-affirm long term management plans.

KNOWLEDGE

Pediatric hospitalists should be able to:
- Discuss the pathophysiology of asthma addressing both bronchoconstrictive and inflammatory components and state how each impacts pharmacologic treatment choices.

- Compare and contrast the pathophysiology of asthma with other common small airway illnesses in children such as bronchiolitis, viral pneumonia with bronchospasm, or chronic lung disease.
- List the differential diagnosis of wheezing for various age groups and delineate the defining features leading to a diagnosis of asthma.
- Summarize evaluation, monitoring, and treatment options for patients with worsening cardiorespiratory status including mental status assessment, capnography, inhaled and intravenous medications, respiratory support and others.
- Describe the signs and symptoms of impending respiratory failure and list criteria for transfer to an intensive care unit.
- Cite the common complications of asthma or asthma treatment, including pneumothorax, atelectasis, lobar collapse, poor cardiac output, dysrhythmias and others.
- State the basic pharmacology, safety profile and potential adverse effects of commonly used medications.
- Discuss the impact of risk factors (such as genetic predisposition and family history) associated chronic co-morbidities (such as atopic dermatitis and allergic rhinitis) and exacerbating factors (such as gastroesophageal reflux and smoke exposure) on morbidity, treatment and prognosis.
- Define asthma groups by symptom severity and frequency based on current classification guidelines.
- Explain the significance of environmental controls and trigger avoidance in minimizing asthma exacerbations.
- Describe the utility of using asthma action plans to both monitor and treat asthma via pulmonary function testing (spirometry and/or peak flow) and proper use of controller and reliever medications.
- Discuss the goals of asthma management, including the maintenance of normal activity levels and pulmonary function, the prevention of chronic symptoms, recurrent exacerbations, and hospitalizations, and the provision of optimal pharmacotherapy while minimizing adverse events.
- Give examples of specific indications for referral to an asthma subspecialist.
- Illustrate why proper coding for asthma is critical to assure proper local resource use, accurate billing, and appropriate national comparisons of asthma data.

SKILLS

Pediatric hospitalists should be able to:
- Correctly diagnose and classify asthma by efficiently performing an accurate history and physical examination.
- Recognize signs and symptoms of serious complications of asthma such as pneumothorax or impending respiratory failure.
- Direct an evidence-based treatment plan for status asthmaticus.
- Order and interpret objective measures of pulmonary function, including peak flow monitoring and spirometry.
- Order and interpret results of basic diagnostic tools such as chest radiograph and blood gas as indicated.
- Order appropriate monitoring and correctly interpret monitor data.
- Provide supplemental oxygen therapy and advanced airway management as necessary.
- Recognize indications for hospital admission and discharge, and for transfer to a higher level of care or tertiary care facility.
- Modify the medication regimen based upon accurate assessment of changes in disease severity.
- Efficiently render care by creating a discharge plan which can be expediently activated when appropriate.
- Consistently initiate patient and family/caregiver asthma education as soon after admission as possible, as appropriate for the clinical context.
- Coordinate care with the primary care provider including discharge medications and instructions, and follow-up plans.
- Complete a written asthma action plan and use it to educate patients and the family/caregiver on trigger avoidance, medication adherence, and disease control.

ATTITUDES

Pediatric hospitalists should be able to:
- Reinforce the role and responsibility of patients and the family/caregiver regarding self-care, recognition of symptoms, and disease management.
- Communicate effectively with patients, the family/caregiver and healthcare providers regarding care plans.

- Engage in a multi-disciplinary approach to the prevention, diagnosis, and treatment of asthma, involving when appropriate, social workers or case managers, respiratory therapists, and subspecialists.
- Collaborate with primary care providers and subspecialists to ensure coordinated longitudinal care for children with asthma.

SYSTEMS ORGANIZATION AND IMPROVEMENT

In order to improve efficiency and quality within their organizations, pediatric hospitalists should:
- Lead, coordinate or participate in local and national initiatives to further the development and implementation of evidence-based clinical guidelines to promote effective resource utilization and improve quality of care for hospitalized children with asthma.
- Work with hospital administrators to implement and utilize performance feedback and quality improvement measures to assess outcomes of instituted guidelines for the management of inpatient asthma.
- Collaborate with primary care providers, subspecialists, social workers, and case managers to ensure a smooth transition to the outpatient setting, and to minimize the need for readmission.

BONE AND JOINT INFECTIONS

INTRODUCTION

Osteomyelitis is a pyogenic infection of the bone or periosteum, whereas septic arthritis is an infection of the joint space itself. These occur in children as a result of hematogenous spread or local invasion after soft tissue infection or trauma. Either site of infection may represent a medical emergency in children. Bone and joint infections are commonly caused by Staphylococcus aureus, Streptococcal species and Salmonella. These infections can occur at any age, with osteomyelitis occurring in as many as 1 in 5000 children every year. Males are nearly twice as likely to be affected compared to females. Prompt recognition and appropriate treatment are essential to reduce the risk of significant complications including permanent bone or cartilage destruction with life-long disability. Pediatric hospitalists are often in the best position to render acute inpatient care and coordinate transition to outpatient care to ensure best outcomes.

KNOWLEDGE

Pediatric hospitalists should be able to:
- Discuss the differential diagnosis of common presenting signs and symptoms of bone and joint infections including swollen joint, limp and bone pain.
- Describe the pathophysiology of osteomyelitis including the most common site of infection in a developing bone.
- Explain the pathophysiologic mechanisms involved in septic arthritis.
- Compare and contrast the varied clinical presentations of bone and soft tissue infections in children of differing ages (infancy to adolescence) and underlying co-morbidities (such as sickle cell disease, immunosuppressed, and others).
- Identify indications for admission to the hospital for children with suspected osteomyelitis and septic arthritis and goals for therapy during the inpatient stay.
- Classify the most likely pathogens based on age, underlying risk factors, and exposures and list appropriate antimicrobial agents for each.
- State relative local antimicrobial resistance rates for the most common organisms and explain the importance of these in prescribing therapy.
- Describe the relative advantages, disadvantages, and local availability of commonly used laboratory (such as C - reactive protein, blood cultures, bone aspirate and other) and radiologic (such as plain film, computed tomography, bone scan, magnetic resonance imaging and other) modalities in the evaluation of bone and joint infections.
- Discuss the role of various services in pain management, such as child life and the acute pain service.
- State the available home care services for children in the area served and explain the role of home care in discharge decision making.
- Define the role of the orthopedist and infectious diseases subspecialists in consultation, co-management, and follow-up care.

- Compare and contrast the expertise, skill sets, and availability of orthopedists with pediatric orthopedists in the local area and list criteria for transfer to a tertiary care center attending to local context.
- List the components of an efficient and effective hospital discharge, including documentation of appropriate clinical improvement, discharge planning completed, antimicrobial therapy duration and monitoring determined, and others.
- Identify aspects of diagnosis and treatment that may impact prognosis.

SKILLS

Pediatric hospitalists should be able to:
- Correctly diagnose osteomyelitis or septic arthritis by efficiently performing an accurate history and physical examination.
- Order appropriate diagnostic studies and correctly interpret study results.
- Develop a cost effective diagnostic work-up for bone and joint infections, including laboratory and radiographic testing.
- Manage pain for children with bone and joint infections.
- Consult appropriate subspecialists in a timely and effective manner.
- Demonstrate competence in placing parenterally inserted central catheters (PICC) or efficiently obtain services for PICC placement.
- Efficiently access and arrange for pediatric home care services as appropriate.
- Coordinate care with subspecialists and the primary care provider and arrange an appropriate transition plan for hospital discharge.

ATTITUDES

Pediatric hospitalists should be able to:
- Communicate effectively with patients, the family/caregiver and healthcare providers regarding findings and care plans.
- Assume responsibility for care as the primary attending or in collaboration with the orthopedic team.

SYSTEMS ORGANIZATION AND IMPROVEMENT

In order to improve efficiency and quality within their organizations, pediatric hospitalists should:
- Lead, coordinate or participate in the development and implementation of cost-effective, safe, evidence-based care pathways to standardize the evaluation and management for hospitalized children with bone and joint infections.
- Work with hospital administration to recruit a multidisciplinary team in the care of children with bone and joint infections that may include nursing, social work, physical therapy, pharmacy and care coordinators.
- Assist in creating systems to evaluate and improve pain management for children hospitalized with bone and joint infections.
- Lead, coordinate or participate in efforts to increase pediatric-specific community health care resources that allow for an efficient transition to outpatient therapy and management after inpatient goals are achieved.

BRONCHIOLITIS

INTRODUCTION

Bronchiolitis is the most common viral lower respiratory illness in young children and infants. It is responsible for hundreds of thousands of outpatient and emergency department visits and nearly 150,000 hospitalizations per year, costing the U.S. healthcare system more than $500 million annually. The most commonly identified etiology of bronchiolitis is respiratory syncytial virus (RSV), however bronchiolitis may be caused by many other viruses, including human metapneumovirus, adenovirus, and influenza. Despite guidelines published by the American Academy of Pediatrics on the diagnosis and management of bronchiolitis, there is significant variation in care of hospitalized patients. Pediatric hospitalists should render evidence-based care that avoids use of unnecessary tests and procedures and improves outcomes.

KNOWLEDGE

Pediatric hospitalists should be able to:
- Compare and contrast the epidemiology and pathogenesis of bronchiolitis with asthma.
- Describe the typical clinical presentation of viral bronchiolitis including wheezing, tachypnea, acute respiratory distress, hypoxia, cough, apnea, and/or nasal obstruction, and give examples of how presentations may vary.
- Review alternate diagnoses which may mimic the presentation of bronchiolitis such as congestive heart failure, previously undiagnosed cyanotic or non-cyanotic congenital heart disease, metabolic acidosis, sepsis, aspiration, and others.
- Identify the risk factors such as prematurity, congenital heart disease, pulmonary disease, immunodeficiency, and environmental smoke exposure that predispose infants and children to severe illness or complications of bronchiolitis.
- State the indications and contraindications for RSV immunoprophylaxis.
- List the indications for hospital admission and cite discharge criteria.
- Discuss indications for ordering viral antigen testing and chest radiographs.
- Compare and contrast initial diagnostic evaluation for febrile infants of various ages presenting with bronchiolitis attending to ages less than 30 days, 31-60 days and others.
- Discuss the evidence regarding beta-agonist and steroid therapy in routine bronchiolitis.
- Discuss the evidence regarding use of supportive measures including suctioning, positioning, enteral versus intravenous fluids and nutrition, and supplemental oxygen.
- Discuss the benefits and potential technical errors associated with use of various non-invasive monitoring modalities including cardiorespiratory, oxygen saturation, and capnography.
- Describe a management strategy for patients with worsening respiratory status including the use of different oxygen delivery systems and methods for positive pressure ventilation.
- Describe a management strategy for patients with worsening respiratory status including use of different oxygen delivery systems and methods for positive pressure ventilation.

SKILLS

Pediatric hospitalists should be able to:
- Correctly diagnose bronchiolitis by efficiently performing an accurate history and physical examination; determining if key features of the disease are present.
- Accurately assess clinical signs of respiratory distress and identify impending respiratory failure.
- Assess nutrition and hydration status and chose appropriate methods to maintain adequate hydration and nutrition.
- Order appropriate monitoring and correctly interpret monitor data.
- Objectively assess the response to any medications trialed and use clinical exam and respiratory scores to determine true efficacy.
- Perform careful reassessments daily and as needed, note changes in clinical status and respond with appropriate actions including discontinuation of ineffective or unnecessary therapies.
- Recognize the indications for escalating level of care and initiate basic ventilatory support if indicated.
- Implement appropriate oxygen weaning strategies, including the use of appropriate oxygen saturation parameters.
- Engage the family/caregiver in assisting with interpreting clinical status changes and in determining care plans.
- Consistently adhere to proper infection control measures.
- Efficiently render care by creating a discharge plan which can be expediently activated when appropriate.

ATTITUDES

Pediatric hospitalists should be able to:
- Educate the family/caregiver on the etiologies and natural history of bronchiolitis, including the importance of hand washing and minimizing environmental exposure in the prevention of infection.
- Discuss with the family/caregiver the importance of supportive care, as well as the limited evidence supporting other interventions.
- Display proactive, engaged behavior regarding proper isolation measures particularly including hand-washing to prevent spread of the etiologic agent in the hospital.

- Educate the family/caregiver regarding the relationship between hospitalization for bronchiolitis and risk of future wheezing based on the most current evidence.
- Collaborate with the primary care provider to ensure a smooth transition to the outpatient setting, and to minimize the need for readmission.

SYSTEMS ORGANIZATION AND IMPROVEMENT

In order to improve efficiency and quality within their organizations, pediatric hospitalists should:
- Collaborate with hospital infection control practitioners to prevent nosocomial infection related to bronchiolitis.
- Partner with community services to educate the public on respiratory infection preventive strategies.
- Work with emergency department physicians to mutually develop and implement evidence-based admission criteria.
- Lead, coordinate or participate in multidisciplinary initiatives to develop, implement, and assess quality outcomes of evidence-based clinical guidelines.

CENTRAL NERVOUS SYSTEM INFECTIONS

INTRODUCTION

Central nervous system (CNS) infections in children vary widely in incidence and severity. Enteroviral meningitis is relatively common and usually resolves without sequelae. In contrast, viral encephalitides and suppurative CNS infections are less common, but are associated with significant mortality and long-term morbidity in survivors. Children with CNS implanted devices are particularly diagnostically challenging. All of these infections require prompt diagnosis and initiation of therapy which may require coordination of care with neurologists, neurosurgeons, infectious diseases, neuroradiologists and other subspecialists for optimal outcomes. Pediatric hospitalists are often in the best position to render both coordinated acute care and transition to outpatient care or rehabilitation facility.

KNOWLEDGE

Pediatric hospitalists should be able to:
- Describe the features of the history (such as back pain, trauma, sinus disease, emesis and others) that suggest CNS infections for varied age groups, including those features that differentiate encephalitis, meningitis, brain abscess, and spinal epidural abscess.
- List the physical examination findings (such as focal neurologic findings, rash, mental status changes and others) that suggest CNS infections for varied age groups, including those features that differentiate encephalitis, meningitis, brain abscess, and spinal epidural abscess.
- List key elements to obtain in the history such as travel, environmental exposures, animal and insect bites, water sources, and explain how each assists with development of a differential diagnosis for potential etiologic pathogens.
- Identify the elements of the history and physical examination that may present in a different manner in patients with underlying co-morbidities such as ventricular shunts/reservoirs, implanted CNS devices, immunosuppressant use, developmental delay and others.
- Compare and contrast the cerebrospinal fluid (CSF) analysis values found in viral, bacterial, atypical bacterial and fungal meningitis, encephalitis, brain abscesses, ventricular infections, and suppurative parameningeal foci.
- Identify conditions that predispose to focal, suppurative CNS infections.
- Discuss the risks, benefits, and indications for lumbar puncture.
- State appropriate microbiologic, virologic, and serologic tests utilized to establish a diagnosis.
- Compare and contrast the value of computed tomography versus magnetic resonance for imaging possible CNS infections of the head, neck, and spine, attending to sedation needs, local availability, radiation exposure, and value of contrast versus non-contrast images.
- Summarize the indications for imaging for meningitis, encephalitis, brain abscess, ventricular infections, and parameningeal infections stating modality of choice for each diagnosis.
- Describe the approach toward initial antimicrobial therapy for CNS infections, attending to age, likely pathogens, and site of infection.
- Explain the importance of CNS drug penetration, microbial drug resistance, and age on initial antimicrobial therapy choice.

- Name the most common significant complications of CNS infections such as fluid and electrolyte imbalance, seizures, and increase intracranial pressure.

SKILLS

Pediatric hospitalists should be able to:
- Elicit key historical data that may distinguish between types of CNS infections.
- Demonstrate proficiency in performing a careful global physical examination to document features to support or refute various infectious etiologies.
- Perform a thorough neurologic examination to identify global or focal neurologic deficits.
- Efficiently and effectively perform a lumbar puncture.
- Determine best patient placement (bed or ward assignment) based on local monitoring and nursing capabilities and patient clinical status.
- Initiate appropriate empiric therapy for CNS infections and modify therapy based on proper interpretation of microbiologic, virologic and serologic data.
- Anticipate, recognize, and manage acute complications of CNS infections.
- Recognize the indications for transfer to higher level of care and effectively coordinate the transfer.
- Obtain and coordinate appropriate consults in a timely manner.
- Identify patients with neurologic sequelae and make appropriate referrals for therapy and rehabilitation services.
- Coordinate care with subspecialists and the primary care provider and arrange an appropriate transition plan for hospital discharge inclusive of therapies, school needs, and psychosocial support.
- Consistently adhere to proper infection control practices.

ATTITUDES

Pediatric hospitalists should be able to:
- Engage consultants in sensitive and clear communications with the family/caregiver regarding potential long term neurologic sequelae as appropriate.
- Realize the impact of the illness on the family/caregiver, and maintain empathy at all times.
- Recognize that the family/caregiver may not assimilate information during times of stress, and that delivering a clear, coherent assessment and plan on repeated occasions may be needed.
- Collaborate with subspecialists and the primary care provider to ensure coordinated longitudinal care for children with CNS infection.
- Collaborate with public health officials when indicated.

SYSTEMS ORGANIZATION AND IMPROVEMENT

In order to improve efficiency and quality within their organizations, pediatric hospitalists should:
- Lead, coordinate or participate in the development and implementation of cost-effective, safe, evidence-based care pathways to standardize the evaluation and management for hospitalized children with CNS infections.
- Collaborate with hospital administration, hospital staff, and others to create a multidisciplinary approach toward care and support for children with CNS infections.
- Work with hospital and community leaders to assure proper services are available for children requiring short and long term support services.

DIABETES MELLITUS

INTRODUCTION

Diabetes mellitus, a disorder of glucose homeostasis, is increasing in incidence and prevalence in pediatrics. Although Type 1 diabetes is more frequently diagnosed in children, there has recently been a significant rise in the incidence of Type 2 diabetes, particularly among adolescents in certain ethnic groups. The increasing incidence of Type 2 diabetes parallels the increasing incidence of obesity in the population. In addition to the medical complications associated with this chronic disease, both forms of diabetes have profound social and emotional impacts on the child. Pediatric hospitalists frequently encounter both children with new-onset diabetes and known diabetics requiring hospitalization because of poor disease control, illness, or elective procedures. Pediatric hospitalists are often in the best position to provide both immediate care for children with diabetes as well as to coordinate care across multiple specialties when necessary.

KNOWLEDGE

Pediatric hospitalists should be able to:
- Compare and contrast the epidemiology and pathophysiology of Type 1 with Type 2 diabetes attending to differences in impairment of glucose regulation and occurrence of ketoacidosis.
- List common alternate causes of hyperglycemia, such as stress, drug, or steroid-induced hyperglycemia and give examples of situations in which insulin administration is indicated.
- Discuss the importance of completing a thorough review of systems and family history and a full physical examination in order to identify polyendocrinopathies.
- Describe the role of obesity in the metabolic syndrome and Type 2 diabetes.
- List and explain the laboratory tests used to determine the type of diabetes, assess glucose control, and identify complications or co-morbidities of diabetes (such as glutamic acid decarboxylase, insulin auto antibodies, islet cell antibodies, hemoglobin A1c, thyroid panel, and celiac panel).
- Describe the initial management of diabetic ketoacidosis (DKA), attending to fluid delivery, electrolyte monitoring, mental status assessments, frequency of repeated blood testing, and appropriate patient placement based on local facility services.
- Define criteria for escalating care in the context of severe acidosis, altered mental status, and effects of electrolyte disturbances.
- Summarize the approach toward management and education after stabilization of DKA.
- Discuss the importance of including cultural and ethnic practices when creating a diabetes management plan.
- Discuss potential complications that may result from treatment, including hypoglycemia and electrolyte imbalances
- Identify the co-morbidities commonly associated with both Type 1 and Type 2 diabetes.
- Describe the different formulations of and delivery systems for insulin.
- Review the principles of carbohydrate counting.
- Discuss short and long-term prognostic factors associated with complications of poor glucose control.

SKILLS

Pediatric hospitalists should be able to:
- Correctly diagnose diabetes and its complications by efficiently performing an accurate history and physical examination, determining if key features of the disease are present.
- Correctly recognize and determine the cause of DKA in the patient with known diabetes by efficiently performing an accurate history and physical examination and ordering appropriate diagnostic tests.
- Order appropriate diagnostic testing for patients with new onset diabetes or diabetes exacerbations.
- Implement an evidence-based treatment plan.
- Correctly order insulin doses and delivery systems (such as continuous infusion, subcutaneous, and others) and other classes of drugs used in the treatment of diabetes.
- Recognize and manage both hyperglycemia and hypoglycemia with particular attention to complications that may arise during treatment.
- Recognize the indications for escalating levels of care and promptly initiate appropriate actions.
- Identify the indications for in hospital consultation and obtain prompt consultation with an endocrinologist or other subspecialist as appropriate.
- Access available support services such as social work, child life, nutrition, and others to ensure a comprehensive management approach.
- Clearly articulate discharge criteria and outpatient long term management strategies for patients and the family/caregiver.
- Coordinate care and education for patients and the family/caregiver with other healthcare providers.
- Coordinate care with subspecialists and the primary care provider and arrange an appropriate transition plan for hospital discharge.

ATTITUDES

Pediatric hospitalists should be able to:
- Communicate effectively with patients maintaining awareness of the unique needs of pre-adolescent and adolescent age groups.
- Discuss the importance of a healthy lifestyle in promoting optimal disease management with patients and the family/caregiver.
- Recognize that acute and chronic psychosocial factors impact the ability of patients and the family/caregiver to appropriately manage the disease.
- Recognize the importance of the multidisciplinary team approach in the management of diabetes in children, including involvement of the primary care provider, endocrinologist, nutritionist, social worker, psychologist, child life, and school representative.
- Maintain awareness of local populations which may have multiple risk factors for diabetes
- Collaborate with subspecialists and the primary care provider to ensure coordinated longitudinal care for children with diabetes.

SYSTEMS ORGANIZATION AND IMPROVEMENT

In order to improve efficiency and quality within their organizations, pediatric hospitalists should:
- Lead, coordinate or participate in the development and implementation of cost-effective, safe, evidence-based care pathways to standardize the evaluation and management for hospitalized children with diabetes.
- Work with hospital administration, hospital staff, subspecialists and community organizations to affect system-wide processes to improve the transition of care from hospital to the ambulatory setting.
- Lead, coordinate or participate in system-wide processes within the hospital to promote therapeutic safety and vigilance in the use of hypoglycemic agents.
- Lead, coordinate or participate in educational events to promote awareness of and familiarity with national guidelines for management strategies, new therapeutic and pharmacologic agents and the use of medical devices to improve and monitor glucose homeostasis.

FAILURE TO THRIVE

INTRODUCTION

Failure to thrive (FTT) is a descriptive term that refers to a child with relative undernutrition and subsequent inadequate growth over time, when compared to other children of similar age, gender, and ethnicity. Several definitions have been proposed based on abnormal anthropometric criteria, but none is uniformly accepted. The etiology of FTT is often multifactorial and results from a complex interplay between psychosocial, behavioral, and physiological factors. Ultimately, this interaction leads to one of three outcomes – inadequate caloric intake (in the setting of normal or excessive metabolic demands), inadequate absorption of calories, or impaired utilization of absorbed calories. FTT is often successfully managed in the outpatient setting. However, hospitalization may be necessary for very complex situations, when a child's safety is in question, or when outpatient management has not been successful. It is estimated that FTT accounts for 1 to 5% of all pediatric hospitalizations. Pediatric hospitalists should use evidence-based approaches to guide evaluation and management, provide leadership for multidisciplinary teams, and coordinate care to optimize outcomes.

KNOWLEDGE

Pediatric hospitalists should be able to:
- Describe the differential diagnosis of FTT for children of varying chronological and developmental ages recognizing that most children with FTT do not have an underlying medical disorder.
- Explain why infants and toddlers are at greater risk for FTT than older children.
- Describe the association between FTT and child abuse and neglect.
- Describe normal growth patterns for children and the sequential effect of undernutrition on weight velocity, height velocity, and head growth.
- Describe the key historical or physical examination findings that may indicate a psychosocial, behavioral, or physiological factor contributing to poor growth.

- Provide indications for admission to the hospital and state criteria for determining the appropriate level of care (ward vs. intensive care unit).
- Describe the goals of hospitalization including stabilization, diagnosis, treatment, observation, and education.
- Discuss the importance of observation of feeding behaviors and recording of nutritional intake over time in the evaluation of FTT.
- State the indications for laboratory, radiographic, or other testing in the evaluation of FTT.
- Discuss the indications for consultation with a pediatric speech or occupational therapist, nutritionist, gastroenterologist or other subspecialist.
- Discuss the need for catch-up calories in FTT, as well as the methods by which to achieve adequate caloric supplementation.
- Define the refeeding syndrome, and describe methods to prevent it or lead to its early detection.
- Discuss potential sequelae of FTT (such as behavioral or developmental abnormalities, increased susceptibility to infections, and others) and list the risk factors for worse outcomes.
- Summarize the literature on the impact of hospitalization on the evaluation, management, and outcomes for FTT.

SKILLS

Pediatric hospitalists should be able to:
- Stabilize patients presenting with metabolic abnormalities, cardiopulmonary compromise, or other urgent problems as a result of dehydration, malnutrition, or an abnormal pathophysiological state.
- Obtain a thorough patient history, including a detailed social, family, dietary and feeding history, attending to markers of abnormal behavioral or psychosocial factors.
- Perform a directed physical examination, including careful measurement of anthropometric data, attending to findings that may indicate an underlying medical condition or child abuse and neglect.
- Correctly utilize standardized growth charts to identify isolated growth abnormalities and to assess the growth pattern over time.
- Directly observe and correctly interpret a feeding session, with attention paid to feeding behavior and the child-caregiver interactions.
- Critically assess the level of evidence and risk/benefit ratio for an expanded diagnostic evaluation.
- Interpret basic tests and identify abnormal findings that require further testing or consultation.
- Correctly calculate caloric needs and adjust feeding regimens to maximize weight gain while avoiding gastrointestinal compromise.
- Correctly identify the need for and efficiently access appropriate consultants and support services needed to provide comprehensive care.
- Coordinate care with subspecialists, the primary care provider and other services and arrange for an appropriate transition plan with detailed follow-up plans for after hospital discharge.

ATTITUDES

Pediatric hospitalists should be able to:
- Consider the concerns of the family/caregiver when obtaining a history, developing a diagnostic approach, and offering anticipatory guidance and management options.
- Provide education to the family/caregiver on FTT, with specific focus on patient-specific underlying diagnoses.
- Communicate effectively with the family/caregiver and healthcare providers regarding findings and care plans.
- Maintain the continuum of care by effectively coordinating the discharge with the primary care provider.

SYSTEMS ORGANIZATION AND IMPROVEMENT

In order to improve efficiency and quality within their organizations, pediatric hospitalists should:
- Coordinate the care of professional staff (including social work, nursing, speech or occupational therapists) and consultants to improve the quality and efficiency of care.
- Work with healthcare providers and community leaders to develop a system for effective and safe transitions of care from the inpatient to outpatient healthcare providers, preserving the multidisciplinary nature of the care team when appropriate.

- Lead, coordinate or participate in efforts to develop evidence-based guidelines for the evaluation and management of FTT in the hospital.

FEVER OF UNKNOWN ORIGIN

INTRODUCTION

Fever is the most common presenting complaint in the pediatric outpatient and emergency room setting. In most cases, the etiology of acute fever is readily discernable. In contrast, fever of unknown origin (FUO) is typically defined as fever of 38.3° C (101° F) or greater of at least 14 days duration, with no apparent cause after a thorough history, physical examination, and intense laboratory evaluation of one-week duration in the outpatient or hospital setting. The differential diagnosis of FUO is very broad, but infection is the most common cause of prolonged fever. Other major etiologic categories include malignancy, rheumatologic conditions, vasculitis syndromes, inflammatory bowel disease, drug fever, and miscellaneous causes. When children require hospitalization for prolonged fever with concern for FUO, pediatric hospitalists should develop a thoughtful, step-wise, and cost-effective approach to diagnosis and management

KNOWLEDGE

Pediatric hospitalists should be able to:
- Discuss the pathophysiologic mechanisms that result in fever.
- List the different methods available for obtaining a temperature and explain common errors associated with each.
- Differentiate serial or prolonged fevers with known etiologies from FUO.
- Describe the differential diagnosis of FUO for children of varying chronological and developmental ages and state the relative prevalence of each etiologic category.
- Identify the common infectious causes of FUO, particularly as they differ by region.
- Describe the key historical features to elicit including details of the fever pattern and course of illness, immunization status, travel and exposure history, and family history.
- Review areas of specific focus when performing the physical examination, including skin and eye findings, lymph nodes, sinuses, liver and spleen size, bone and joint exam, and neurobehavioral state.
- List common initial laboratory tests for FUO, recognizing the utility, sensitivity and specificity of diagnostic tests as well as local availability and turnaround times.
- Describe the indications for and goals of hospitalization and explain the role of close observation without treatment and daily physical examination.
- Discuss the benefits, risks, and potential complications of empiric antibiotic treatment.
- Compare and contrast the mechanisms of action and modifying effect on systemic symptoms of anti-pyretics versus anti-inflammatory agents noting common side effects.
- Identify indications for consultation with a subspecialist.
- Summarize the diagnostic value of commonly used "second or third tier" testing (such as bone scan, bone marrow aspiration/biopsy, repeated blood cultures with fever, and others) where initial testing and observation is non-diagnostic.

SKILLS

Pediatric hospitalists should be able to:
- Obtain a thorough fever history, including duration, height, pattern, associated signs and symptoms, and response to anti-pyretics.
- Obtain a complete medical history, including signs and symptoms, immunization status, travel history, exposure history (such as animals, tick bites, consumption of raw foods or contaminated water, sick contacts, and others), and family history.
- Perform a comprehensive physical examination.
- Perform careful reassessments daily and as needed, note changes in clinical status and test results and respond with appropriate actions.
- Access and comprehensively review all relevant prior records.

- Correctly interpret the results of laboratory or radiological tests performed, engaging subspecialists as needed for interpretation.
- Conduct a cost-effective and evidence-based evaluation plan, avoiding unnecessary repeat testing.
- Correctly order laboratory studies with appropriate detail to ensure specimens are correctly collected and handled.
- Appropriately differentiate when to continue inpatient versus outpatient diagnostic evaluation in the face of persistent fever and pending test results.
- Formulate appropriate treatment plans for the presumptive or confirmed diagnosis when indicated.
- Access and consult subspecialists when indicated.
- Create an effective discharge plan including specific expectations for home observation for fever and other symptoms.

ATTITUDES

Pediatric hospitalists should be able to:
- Communicate effectively with the primary care provider regarding the evaluation and treatment conducted in and out of the hospital.
- Realize the significant stress placed on the family/caregiver when the diagnosis is unclear and multiple healthcare providers are involved in care.
- Educate patients and the family/caregiver regarding the importance of observation and the need for a thoughtful, step-wise approach to the diagnosis and potential treatment plan.
- Recognize the important role pediatric hospitalists play in coordination of care given the often multiple, potentially invasive testing that may be necessary.
- Collaborate with subspecialists and the primary care provider to ensure coordinated longitudinal care for children with FUO as appropriate.

SYSTEMS ORGANIZATION AND IMPROVEMENT

In order to improve efficiency and quality within their organizations, pediatric hospitalists should:
- Lead, coordinate or participate in multidisciplinary initiatives to streamline the admission process to assure smooth, complete transmission of or access to outpatient medical information.
- Promote the effective use of hospital resources by adhering to a targeted, step-wise, and evidence-based approach to diagnosis and management.
- Lead, coordinate or participate in multidisciplinary teams to facilitate discharge planning, including a safe transition from inpatient to outpatient healthcare providers.

GASTROENTERITIS

INTRODUCTION

Gastroenteritis is one of the most common diseases of childhood, accounting for thousands of hospital admissions each year. Admission to the hospital can be prevented in most cases with appropriate use of oral rehydration. Although uncommon in developed countries, morbidity and mortality can occur, especially among hospitalized infants with severe dehydration, electrolyte abnormalities, sepsis or malnutrition. Misdiagnosis of gastroenteritis may occur, particularly when vomiting is the predominant symptom, which can lead to inappropriate treatment for potentially life threatening conditions. Pediatric hospitalists routinely encounter patients with gastroenteritis and should provide immediate medical care in an efficient and effective manner.

KNOWLEDGE

Pediatric hospitalists should be able to:
- Review the elements of the history which are pertinent to obtain, such as travel, immunization status, water source, daycare attendance, food sources and methods of preparation and others.
- Describe the elements of the physical examination that aid in supporting or refuting the diagnosis.

- Cite critical medical (such as diabetic ketoacidosis, CNS infection or injury, malabsorption, toxic ingestion, inborn errors of metabolism, and others) and surgical (such as bowel obstruction, testicular/ovarian torsion, and others) differential diagnoses to consider and describe the key history and physical examination findings of each, attending to differences by age.
- Compare and contrast the differential diagnoses of isolated emesis versus emesis with diarrhea.
- Describe the differences in approach toward diagnosis and treatment for patients with underlying co-morbidities or receiving treatments which may affect potential pathogens.
- List the common etiologies for gastroenteritis depending upon geographic location and age.
- Summarize the literature on gastroenteritis epidemiology, immunizations, and global health impact.
- Describe the epidemiologic factors associated with different pathogens, such as close contact with other symptomatic individuals, intake of contaminated food or water, case clustering, and recent travel to an endemic area.
- Compare and contrast clinical findings which are more suggestive of viral, bacterial, and parasitic gastroenteritis.
- Discuss the role of infection control in the hospital, as well as public health reporting mandates.
- List the indications for diagnostic laboratory tests, including stool, blood, and urine studies, attending to age groups, predictive value of tests, and cost-effectiveness.
- Describe the role of oral rehydration solutions in the treatment of dehydration related to gastroenteritis.
- List the indications for hospital admission, including the need for intravenous fluids, correction of fluid, electrolyte and acid base disturbances, close clinical monitoring and/or further diagnostic evaluation.

SKILLS

Pediatric hospitalists should be able to:
- Correctly diagnose gastroenteritis by efficiently performing an accurate history and physical examination, determining if key features of the disease are present.
- Recognize and correctly manage dehydration, fluid, electrolyte and acid base derangements.
- Recognize and assess patients for complications of gastroenteritis such as sepsis, significant ileus, and hemolytic uremic syndrome.
- Identify findings of and appropriately evaluate patients for alternative conditions.
- Identify and appropriately treat patients at risk for unusual pathogens.
- Direct a cost-effective and evidence-based evaluation and treatment plan, especially with regard to laboratory studies, antibiotics, and oral or intravenous fluid resuscitation.
- Consistently adhere to infection control practices.
- Efficiently render care by creating a discharge plan which can be expediently activated when appropriate.

ATTITUDES

Pediatric hospitalists should be able to:
- Educate the family/caregiver on infection control practices to decrease pathogen transmission.
- Ensure coordination of care for diagnostic tests and treatment between subspecialists.
- Realize the importance of educating the family/caregiver on the natural course of disease to manage expectations for improvement.
- Role model and advocate for strict adherence to infection control practices.
- Communicate effectively with patients, the family/caregiver, and healthcare providers regarding findings, care plans, and anticipated health needs after discharge.

SYSTEMS ORGANIZATION AND IMPROVEMENT

In order to improve efficiency and quality within their organizations, pediatric hospitalists should:
- Lead, coordinate or participate in the development and implementation of cost-effective, safe, evidence-based care pathways to standardize the evaluation and management for hospitalized children with gastroenteritis.
- Work with hospital administration to create and sustain a process to follow up on laboratory tests pending at discharge.

- Collaborate with institutional infection control practitioners to improve processes to prevent nosocomial infection related to gastroenteritis.
- Work with hospital and community leaders to assure consistent public health reporting of appropriate infections and response to trends.

KAWASAKI DISEASE

INTRODUCTION

Kawasaki Disease (KD), also known as mucocutaneous lymph node syndrome, is a multisystem inflammatory disease of childhood. It most commonly presents in children under the age of two, however has been seen up to 12 years of age. Diagnosis can be difficult, as the classic signs and symptoms may not all manifest and the presentation may mimic other causes of fever and rash. Although many organs may be affected, those related to the cardiac system are the most concerning and persistent. Coronary aneurysms have been reported to occur in up to 20% of untreated children with KD. If diagnosed and treated promptly, the cardiac complications can be reduced. Therefore, it is important that pediatric hospitalists have a complete understanding of the diagnostic criteria and treatment of KD.

KNOWLEDGE

Pediatric hospitalists should be able to:
- Discuss current established criteria and guidelines for diagnosis and treatment.
- Define incomplete KD and note age groups in which this is more common.
- List the broad categories of alternate diagnoses, and give examples from each.
- Discuss the appropriate laboratory and imaging studies that aid in diagnosis.
- Explain the pathophysiology of the disease, including the current understanding of development and manifestation of cardiac complications.
- Define refractory KD and the list factors that indicate the need for further treatment.
- Describe current best practice treatments, including approach toward persistent fever.
- Compare and contrast the risks, benefits, and side effects of available treatments such as immunoglobulin, steroids, anti-platelet medications and immunomodulators.
- Cite risk factors associated with increased cardiac complications.
- Discuss the immediate and long term follow-up needed including impact, if any, on physical activity and sports participation.
- List appropriate discharge criteria for KD.

SKILLS

Pediatric hospitalists should be able to:
- Correctly diagnose KD by efficiently performing an accurate history and physical examination, determining if key features of the disease are present.
- Promptly consult appropriate subspecialists to assist in evaluation and treatment.
- Correctly interpret laboratory and imaging results.
- Recognize features of alternate diagnoses and order relevant diagnostic studies as indicated.
- Perform careful reassessments daily and as needed, note changes in clinical status and respond with appropriate actions.
- Initiate prompt treatment once the diagnosis is established.
- Anticipate and treat complications and side effects of instituted therapies.
- Identify treatment failure and institute appropriate repeat or alternate therapy.
- Demonstrate basic proficiency in reading electrocardiograms.
- Coordinate care with subspecialists and the primary care provider, and arrange an appropriate transition and follow-up plans for after hospital discharge.

ATTITUDES

Pediatric hospitalists should be able to:
- Communicate effectively with patients, the family/caregiver, and other healthcare providers regarding findings and care plans.

- Educate patients and the family/caregiver on the natural course of disease.
- Collaborate with subspecialists and the primary care provider to ensure coordinated longitudinal care for children with KD.

SYSTEMS ORGANIZATION AND IMPROVEMENT

In order to improve efficiency and quality within their organizations, pediatric hospitalists should:
- Lead, coordinate or participate in early multidisciplinary care to promote efficient diagnosis, treatment and discharge of patients with KD.
- Work with hospital staff and subspecialists to educate other healthcare providers regarding the diagnosis and treatment of KD.
- Lead, coordinate or participate in community education efforts regarding KD.

NEONATAL FEVER

INTRODUCTION

Fever in a neonate ($\leq$ 28 days of age) is defined as a rectal temperature above 38°C, and may occur in 20% of neonates admitted to the hospital. Approximately 10% of neonates with fever have a serious bacterial infection. However, some neonates with serious bacterial infection present with hypothermia, usually defined as a rectal temperature below 36.5°C. Infection in neonates often occurs as a result of both a naïve immune system and exposure to pathogenic bacteria during delivery, although pathogens acquired in the postnatal period are also possible. Serious bacterial infections in neonates are most predominant in the renal, pulmonary, central nervous, and blood systems. The prevalence of each varies by age and gender. Neonates may also develop serious illness when be exposed to viral infections, especially herpes simplex virus (HSV). In febrile neonates without a clear source of illness, distinguishing between those with self-limiting versus life-threatening infection is challenging. Well-appearing infants over 28 days of age may be managed without hospitalization in selected circumstances. However, more conservative inpatient evaluation, monitoring, and management of neonates younger than 28 days of age with abnormal temperature is currently standard. Pediatric hospitalists should render evidence-based care for these neonates.

KNOWLEDGE

Pediatric hospitalists should be able to:
- Define hypothermia and hyperthermia in neonates and describe how to correctly obtain a temperature using a variety of modalities.
- Discuss the basic mechanisms of temperature regulation in neonates.
- Compare and contrast basic immune maturity differences in neonates versus older infants.
- Delineate the elements of the history (such as birth history, perinatal exposures, maternal infections and others) and physical examination (such as skin lesions, neurobehavioral exam and others) that aid in determining a diagnosis.
- Describe the differential diagnosis of neonatal sepsis and discuss how other potentially serious illnesses, such as inborn error of metabolism, may mimic its presentation.
- List the organisms which are responsible for serious bacterial infection in neonates, including the types of infections they cause and the relative prevalence of each.
- Review the approach toward evaluation in the preterm infant, attending to extent of prematurity and neonatal intensive care course.
- Compare and contrast the signs and symptoms more suggestive of bacterial versus viral illnesses.
- Distinguish between the current standard laboratory evaluation for neonates with that for older infants, using current literature for reference.
- Describe the role of viral testing, including interpretation of frequencies of disease, co-infections with bacterial disease, local turnaround time, and predictive value of testing.
- Summarize the approach to empiric antimicrobial therapy and give examples of situations warranting expanded antimicrobial coverage.

SKILLS

Pediatric hospitalists should be able to:
- Obtain a complete history, including pregnancy and birth history, with particular attention paid to prenatal laboratory screening and the use of antibiotic prophylaxis prior to delivery.
- Perform a comprehensive physical examination, with attention paid to signs and symptoms that may indicate a source of infection or signify severe illness.
- Accurately perform, supervise, or direct basic procedures to obtain specimens, including venipuncture, bladder catheterization, lumbar puncture, and placement of intravenous access.
- Interpret the results of laboratory evaluations efficiently and adjust the differential diagnosis and plan of care accordingly.
- Select appropriate empiric antimicrobial coverage in an evidence-based manner.
- Perform careful reassessments daily and as needed, note changes in clinical status and respond with appropriate actions.
- Efficiently render care by creating a discharge plan which can be expediently activated when appropriate.

ATTITUDES

Pediatric hospitalists should be able to:
- Elicit and allay the concerns of the family/caregiver, educating them regarding the importance of a thorough evaluation for the source of infection and the need for empiric antimicrobial therapy.
- Communicate effectively with the family/caregiver and healthcare providers regarding findings and care plans.
- Educate the family/caregiver about the final diagnosis, clearly explaining the value of negative test results if applicable.
- Recognize the significance of performing invasive procedures on a neonate from the family/caregiver perspective, maintaining empathy when discussing the risks and benefits of necessary procedures.
- Assure an effective and safe discharge by communicating and coordinating effectively with the primary care provider.

SYSTEMS ORGANIZATION AND IMPROVEMENT

In order to improve efficiency and quality within their organizations, pediatric hospitalists should:
- Lead, coordinate or participate in the development and implementation of cost-effective, safe, evidence-based care pathways to standardize the evaluation and management of hospitalized neonates with fever.
- Lead, coordinate or participate in efforts to develop institutional guidelines for the judicious use of antimicrobials in neonates with fever.

NEONATAL JAUNDICE

INTRODUCTION

Jaundice due to unconjugated hyperbilirubinemia is the most common complication of the normal newborn period and occurs in nearly 50% of normal term newborns. Physiologic jaundice occurs as serum bilirubin rises from 1.5mg/dL in cord blood to 6 mg/dL by day 3 of life, followed by a subsequent decline to normal (less than 1 mg/dL) by day 10-12 of life. Physiologic jaundice is a normal process and does not cause morbidity but must be distinguished from pathologic jaundice. Pathologic jaundice can be due to a number of underlying etiologies and may present when there is an onset of clinical jaundice at less than 24 hours of life, the rate of rise of bilirubin is greater than 0.5mg/dL per hour, the serum bilirubin concentration is greater than 20 mg/dL, or the direct (conjugated) bilirubin level is either greater than 2mg/dL or more than 10% of the total bilirubin concentration. Failure to recognize severe hyperbilirubinemia and pathologic jaundice may result in severe morbidity, including bilirubin encephalopathy (kernicterus). Pediatric hospitalists are often asked to provide consultation regarding necessity for admission as well as render inpatient care, and must be knowledgeable about diagnosis and treatment of neonatal jaundice

KNOWLEDGE

Pediatric hospitalists should be able to:
- Describe the physiology of bilirubin production and metabolism including the pathophysiology that leads to jaundice.

- Compare and contrast the features that distinguish pathologic jaundice from physiologic jaundice.
- List the elements of the birth and family histories and review of systems which may aid in determining the etiology of the jaundice.
- Cite the physical examination findings which may support a potential underlying diagnosis attending to skin, abdominal, dysmorphic features and others.
- Discuss risk factors for pathologic jaundice such as prematurity and sepsis.
- Describe the differential diagnosis of direct and indirect hyperbilirubinemia attending to inborn error of metabolism, sepsis, anatomic defects, hemolytic diseases, and others.
- Compare and contrast the pathophysiology and epidemiology breast milk jaundice versus breastfeeding jaundice.
- Review the pathophysiology involved in development of kernicterus including associated factors affecting the blood-brain barrier such as acidosis and prematurity.
- Review the approach toward diagnosis including commonly performed laboratory tests.
- Describe the use of diagnostic imaging in evaluating direct hyperbilirubinemia.
- Explain the current national recommendations for the management of hyperbilirubinemia in the newborn.

SKILLS

Pediatric hospitalists should be able to:
- Recognize jaundice during a newborn physical examination.
- Accurately obtain information from the newborn and maternal histories.
- Perform a comprehensive exam, eliciting findings to support potential underlying diagnoses.
- Correctly order and interpret bilirubin results based on risk factors for developing kernicterus.
- Correctly order and interpret other studies to diagnose underlying conditions.
- Recognize indications for initiating, continuing and discontinuing phototherapy and/or exchange transfusion.
- Efficiently obtain appropriate consultative services for infants with cholestatic jaundice or possible pathologic underlying condition.
- Identify neonates requiring a higher level of care and efficiently coordinate transfer.
- Perform careful reassessments daily and as needed, note changes in clinical status and respond with appropriate actions.
- Efficiently render care by creating a discharge plan that includes an efficient and comprehensive hand-off communication with specific outpatient follow-up needs such as weight checks and repeat lab testing as appropriate.

ATTITUDES

Pediatric hospitalists should be able to:
- Educate the family/caregiver and other professional staff regarding the risks, evaluation and therapies available for hyperbilirubinemia.
- Coordinate discharge plans with the primary care provider and home care agencies as appropriate.

SYSTEMS ORGANIZATION AND IMPROVEMENT

In order to improve efficiency and quality within their organizations, pediatric hospitalists should:
- Lead, coordinate or participate in the development and implementation of cost-effective, safe, evidence-based care pathways to standardize the evaluation and management of hospitalized neonates with jaundice.
- Lead, coordinate or participate in education programs for the family/caregiver and the community to increase awareness of evidence-based guidelines and strategies to reduce admission rates.

PNEUMONIA

INTRODUCTION

Lower respiratory tract infections cause substantial morbidity and mortality in the pediatric population. Worldwide, an estimated 4 million children die from pneumonia each year, with higher mortality rates seen in developing countries. In the United States, pneumonia accounts for up to 1 in 5 pediatric hospitalizations. Pneumonia is commonly caused by a viral infection, especially in children less than 2 years of age. Despite high rates of viral disease in young children, bacterial co-infection is common. Non-viral etiologies for pneumonia differ based upon age and underlying risk factors resulting in the need to tailor antimicrobials appropriately. Surgical intervention may be required when pneumonia is complicated by pleural effusion or abscess. Pediatric hospitalists are the attending of record, coordinate subspecialty care when necessary, and are often in the best position to lead quality improvement initiatives to optimize pneumonia care.

KNOWLEDGE

Pediatric hospitalists should be able to:
- Describe the key features of the history and physical examination that support or refute the diagnosis of pneumonia.
- Discuss the variations in clinical presentation that may accompany chronic health conditions of childhood, such as cystic fibrosis, chronic lung disease, congenital heart disease, immunodeficiency, and others.
- Review alternate diagnoses which may mimic the presentation of pneumonia including anatomic defects, systemic diseases, heart failure, and others.
- Provide indications for hospital admission and determine the appropriate level of care.
- List common bacterial, atypical bacterial, and viral organisms causing pneumonia and state how these differ based on age.
- Name other causes of infectious and non-infectious pneumonias such as lipoid, inhalation pneumonitis, aspiration, and others.
- Discuss the influence of national immunization practices and antimicrobial use on predominant organisms and resistance patterns.
- Describe local resistance patterns for predominant infectious organisms.
- Discuss the benefits and limitations of radiography and laboratory evaluation in the diagnosis of pneumonia.
- Describe common complications seen with pneumonia and list co-morbidities or infectious etiologies associated with higher risk for each.
- Describe the indications and options for surgical intervention in patients with complicated pneumonia.
- Summarize goals for hospital discharge attending to symptoms, oxygenation saturation, hydration, and family/caregiver needs, and outpatient management plans.

SKILLS

Pediatric hospitalists should be able to:
- Correctly diagnose pneumonia by efficiently performing an accurate history and physical examination, determining if key features of the disease are present.
- Order appropriate laboratory and radiographic tests to guide treatment and ensure proper isolation.
- Direct an evidence-based treatment plan, including cardio-respiratory monitoring, oxygen supplementation, and appropriately selected antibiotic therapy as indicated.
- Accurately interpret chest radiographs and distinguishing between consolidation, effusion, mass, and other presentations.
- Perform careful reassessments daily and as needed, note changes in clinical status, and respond with appropriate actions.
- Correctly determine when consultation with a surgeon or other subspecialist or a transfer to a higher level of care is indicated.
- Identify patients requiring extended evaluation for underlying anatomic or systemic disease.
- Coordinate discharge efficiently and effectively with patients, family/caregiver, subspecialists, and the primary care provider including home care needs and follow-up as appropriate.
- Create a comprehensive discharge plan including home care as appropriate.

ATTITUDES

Pediatric hospitalists should be able to:
- Role model and advocate for strict adherence to infection control practices and educate the family/caregiver regarding measures such as handwashing to reduce the spread of infection.

- Communicate effectively with patients, the family/caregiver and healthcare providers regarding findings and care plans.
- Collaborate with subspecialists to render safe and efficient treatment.
- Realize the importance of antimicrobial stewardship and consistently modify prescribing practice to reflect best practices attending to local resistance patterns.

SYSTEMS ORGANIZATION AND IMPROVEMENT

In order to improve efficiency and quality within their organizations, pediatric hospitalists should:
- Work with hospital, community, and infectious disease experts to develop and sustain local communications regarding resistance pattern changes.
- Lead, coordinate or participate in the development and implementation of cost-effective, safe, evidence-based care pathways to standardize the evaluation and management of hospitalized children with pneumonia.

RESPIRATORY FAILURE

INTRODUCTION

Respiratory failure is defined by the inability to provide adequate gas exchange, resulting in ineffective alveolar ventilation and/or oxygenation. The respiratory system includes the upper and lower airways, central and peripheral control mechanisms, nerves and muscles. The differential diagnosis for respiratory failure in children is extensive; failure may stem from any portion of the respiratory system. Children with respiratory conditions are frequently hospitalized and may deteriorate, requiring initiation of rapid response teams or transfer to the critical care unit. Pediatric hospitalists frequently encounter children with conditions affecting the respiratory system, and should be able to recognize and treat those who progress to respiratory failure.

KNOWLEDGE

Pediatric hospitalists should be able to:
- Describe the basic components of the respiratory system, including the upper and lower airways, the central and peripheral regulation systems, peripheral nerves, accessory muscles and diaphragm.
- Discuss the basic principles of respiratory physiology such as the alveolar gas equation, minute ventilation, ventilation-perfusion mismatch, alveolar-arterial gradient, and others.
- Explain the role of the diaphragm and chest wall compliance in development of respiratory failure.
- List causes of poor respiratory muscle function, attending to age, neuromuscular disorders, central nervous system dysfunction, nerve injury, and others.
- Review the anatomy of the upper airway and discuss why progression to respiratory failure can be rapid in young children.
- Describe the differential diagnosis of respiratory distress for children of varying chronological and developmental ages.
- State risk factors and diagnostic categories at higher risk for respiratory failure, attending to acute exposures or events and underlying co-morbidities.
- Summarize the modalities commonly available to support the airway and breathing in children with worsening respiratory distress, such as nasopharyngeal or oropharyngeal airways, bag-valve-mask ventilation, and endotracheal intubation.
- Describe complications due to endotracheal intubation, and state strategies to reduce these risks.
- Summarize evaluation, monitoring, and treatment options for patients with worsening respiratory status including mental status assessment, capnography, medications, respiratory support and others.
- Describe the signs and symptoms of impending respiratory failure and list criteria for transfer to an intensive care unit.

SKILLS

Pediatric hospitalists should be able to:
- Recognize early warning signs of acute respiratory distress and institute corrective actions to avert further deterioration.

- Efficiently stabilize the airway, using effective non-invasive and invasive airway management techniques in collaboration with other services as appropriate.
- Identify patients with risk factors for progression to respiratory failure and assure proper monitoring and patient placement.
- Recognize signs of impending respiratory failure and transfer patients to a critical care unit in an efficient and safe manner.
- Appropriately order, and interpret oxygenation and ventilation testing results.
- Order appropriate monitoring and correctly interpret monitor data.
- Correctly diagnose and initiate medical management for systemic causes of respiratory failure.
- Demonstrate proficiency in basic management of patients with chronic respiratory support needs.
- Identify patients requiring subspecialty care and obtain timely consults.

ATTITUDES

Pediatric hospitalists should be able to:
- Collaborate with patients, the family/caregiver, hospital staff, and subspecialists to ensure coordinated hospital care for children with conditions at risk for respiratory failure.
- Provide consultation for healthcare providers in community ambulatory or inpatient settings to ensure proper patient placement and transport of patients to higher acuity settings as needed.

SYSTEMS ORGANIZATION AND IMPROVEMENT

In order to improve efficiency and quality within their organizations, pediatric hospitalists should:
- Work with hospital administration, hospital staff, subspecialists, and others to develop, implement, and assess outcomes of intervention strategies (rapid response, early warning) for hospitalized patients with deterioration in respiratory status in order to prevent adverse outcomes.
- Lead, coordinate or participate in creating educational programs for the family/caregiver, hospital staff, and other healthcare providers regarding recognition of signs and symptoms of respiratory distress in children, particularly those at higher risk for respiratory failure.

SEIZURES

INTRODUCTION

Seizures are the most common neurologic disorder of childhood. It is estimated that approximately 5% of all children will have at least one seizure before the age of 20. The prevalence of epilepsy, or recurrent unprovoked seizures, is about 0.5% in children. Seizures may range from self-limited to life-threatening events. Status epilepticus is the condition of prolonged seizure activity. Optimal management of seizures not only includes identification of the underlying cause and initiation of appropriate anticonvulsant therapy or other treatments, but also the maintenance and management of an adequate airway and circulation. Pediatric hospitalists frequently encounter patients with active seizures and underlying seizure disorders, and should render both acute care and coordination of multidisciplinary care to the ambulatory setting.

KNOWLEDGE

Pediatric hospitalists should be able to:
- Describe and distinguish between the various manifestations of seizure activity including involuntary motor activity, alterations of consciousness, behavior changes, disturbances of sensation and autonomic dysfunction.
- Classify seizures using appropriate descriptive terms such as generalized, partial, simple and complex.
- Discuss the pathophysiology of seizure activity.
- Review alternate diagnoses which may mimic the presentation of seizures including behavioral abnormalities, movement disorders, conversion disorders and others.
- Compare and contrast distinguishing features of seizures versus other paroxysmal events.
- List the various etiologies of seizures attending to both acute (such as electrolyte imbalance, infection, toxins, trauma and others) and chronic (such as central nervous system malformations, metabolic diseases, and others) causes.

- List the most common etiologies of seizures in various age groups such as the neonate, infant, preschool aged, school aged, and adolescent.
- Define "simple" and "complex" febrile seizures and discuss evaluation, treatment, prognosis, and indications for admission.
- State the common complications associated with seizures and status epilepticus.
- Discuss indications for hospitalization or transfer to a tertiary care facility.
- Discuss indications for transfer to an intensive care unit.
- Review the goals of inpatient diagnostic evaluation and therapy.
- Compare and contrast commonly used anti-epileptic drugs and therapies attending to treatments for specific seizure types, adverse drug events, and ease of use.
- Compare and contrast the risk and benefits of commonly used imaging modalities.
- List the indications for subspecialty consultation.
- Review the management of status epilepticus, including stabilization, testing, monitoring, and patient placement.
- Summarize the risks for readmission, attending to medication management (dosing, availability, pharmacokinetics, and side effect profiles), compliance, and changes in disease state.

SKILLS

Pediatric hospitalists should be able to:
- Correctly diagnose seizures by efficiently performing an accurate history and physical examination with particular focus on the neurologic exam.
- Accurately order appropriate laboratory and radiographic evaluations to identify the etiology of the seizure and potential underlying disorders.
- Interpret laboratory studies including drug levels and make therapy adjustments based on results.
- Order appropriate studies for patients with chronic seizure disorders, avoiding unnecessary duplication of testing and radiation exposure.
- Identify and efficiently treat the cause of the seizure where appropriate.
- Identify status epilepticus and initiate appropriate evidence-based treatment.
- Recognize complications due to seizures and institute appropriate cardiorespiratory support as needed.
- Identify patients at increased risk for seizure recurrence or morbidity and ensures appropriate monitoring and treatment.
- Obtain appropriate consults efficiently.
- Create a comprehensive evaluation and management plan addressing the unique needs of patients and the family/caregiver.
- Anticipate, monitor for, identify, and treat potential side effects of treatment.
- Recognize and efficiently transfer patients requiring higher level of care.

ATTITUDES

Pediatric hospitalists should be able to:
- Communicate effectively with patients, the family/caregiver, hospital staff, subspecialists and primary care provider regarding the reasons for diagnostic testing and therapy choices.
- Recognize the role of patient and family/caregiver education in improving compliance with treatment and follow-up.
- Educate the family/caregiver regarding outcomes of febrile seizures including the risk of the child developing a seizure disorder.
- Collaborate with subspecialists and the primary care provider to ensure coordinated longitudinal care for children with seizure disorders.

SYSTEMS ORGANIZATION AND IMPROVEMENT

In order to improve efficiency and quality within their organizations, pediatric hospitalists should:
- Lead, coordinate or participate in the development and implementation of cost-effective safe, evidence-based care pathways to standardize the evaluation and management of hospitalized children with seizures and status epilepticus.

- Collaborate with hospital administration and community partners to develop and sustain referral networks for both transport and subpsecialty services for children with seizures and chronic seizure disorders.
- Collaborate with primary care providers, subspecialists and other healthcare providers to create effective discharge plans that reduce the likelihood of readmission.

SHOCK

INTRODUCTION

Early recognition and treatment of shock is imperative in improving the outcomes of critically ill children. The American Heart Association categorizes shock into four basic forms: hypovolemic, distributive, cardiogenic, and obstructive. Shock results from inadequate tissue perfusion to support metabolic demands. This may be caused by an inadequate supply of oxygen to the tissues or an increased demand of the tissues for oxygen. As a result, cellular hypoxia, anaerobic metabolism, and dysregulation result in irreversible cell damage and death. Pediatric hospitalists often encounter children with all forms of shock and should be adept at recognition and basic management of shock to improve outcomes.

KNOWLEDGE

Pediatric hospitalists should be able to:
- Discuss the pathophysiology of tissue hypoxia including hypoxemia, anemia, and ischemia.
- Describe the components of tissue oxygen delivery, focusing on cardiac output.
- Describe common diseases and conditions associated with the four forms of shock.
- Compare and contrast the presenting signs and symptoms of the four forms of shock, attending to differences in heart rate, blood pressure, pulses and peripheral perfusion, mental status, and urine output.
- Discuss compensatory mechanisms of early shock including increased heart rate, stroke volume, and vascular smooth muscle tone.
- List indications for chronotropic, inotropic, and blood pressure support and describe the mechanisms of action for these classes of medications.
- State the commonly performed diagnostic studies (such as lab, radiographic, and other) which aid in determining the extent or form of shock.
- Summarize the approach toward stabilization of each form of shock.

SKILLS

Pediatric hospitalists should be able to:
- Perform an initial rapid assessment using Pediatric Advanced Life Support skills.
- Recognize signs of early shock and respond with appropriate actions.
- Appropriately order and correctly interpret results of common studies to determine the extent of shock such as complete blood count, chemistries, blood gas, radiography and others.
- Appropriately order and correctly interpret results of studies to determine the cause of shock and respond with appropriate actions.
- Order appropriate monitoring and correctly interpret monitor data.
- Correctly recognize cardiomegaly and other signs of congestive heart failure on chest radiograph.
- Correctly identify the form of shock from a focused history, physical examination and initial diagnostic studies.
- Initiate appropriate interventions based on the form of shock.
- Facilitate effective transfer to a tertiary care center or intensive care setting when appropriate.

ATTITUDES

Pediatric hospitalists should be able to:
- Communicate effectively with emergency room and intensive care staff to ensure appropriate care for patients in shock.

- Listen effectively and respond to concerns of the family/caregiver and healthcare providers regarding changes in physiologic parameters including vital signs, mental status, physical examination, and urine output.
- Provide family/caregiver support and education on the nuances and complexities of the various forms of shock and the importance of careful monitoring and evaluation.

SYSTEMS ORGANIZATION AND IMPROVEMENT

In order to improve efficiency and quality within their organizations, pediatric hospitalists should:
- Work with hospital administration, hospital staff, subspecialists, and other services to advocate for an educational program for healthcare providers on the importance of early recognition of shock to prevent end-organ failure and death.
- Lead, coordinate or participate in the development and implementation of rapid response systems to assist in recognition and stabilization of early shock.
- Collaborate with hospital administration and community partners to develop and sustain local AHA Pediatric Life Support classes where descriptions and case scenarios provide a comprehensive knowledge base and intervention plan for various types of shock.
- Lead, coordinate or participate in efforts to partner with simulation centers to assist in acquiring skill sets needed for appropriate recognition and intervention for children in shock.

SICKLE CELL DISEASE

INTRODUCTION

Sickle cell disease is the most common autosomal recessive disease in African American individuals. It occurs in 1 in 625 live births to African-American couples. While it is most common in African Americans, it also occurs in individuals of Hispanic, Arabic, Native American and Caucasian heritage. Sickle cell disease results from a single base-pair substitution of thymine for adenine resulting in valine instead of glutamine in the sixth position of the Beta-globin molecule. Sickle cell disease results when this substitution occurs in a homozygous state. Less severe forms occur when the heterozygote state is combined with a second variant Beta-globin chain such as hemoglobin C or Beta⁰-thalassemia. Clinical manifestations result from polymerization of the abnormal hemoglobin and "sickling" of the red cells. The clinical manifestations most important to pediatric hospitalists include recurrent and chronic pain from dactylitis and vaso-occlusive crises, acute chest syndrome, increased susceptibility to infections, aplastic crisis, splenic sequestration, cerebral vascular accidents and priapism. Pediatric hospitalists commonly encounter patients with known or suspected sickle cell disease and care for the various complications associated with the disease.

KNOWLEDGE

Pediatric hospitalists should be able to:
- Review the genetics and pathophysiology underlying the variants of sickle cell disease and their complications.
- Compare and contrast common sickle crisis presentations by age group.
- Explain the impact of newborn screening on preventative care.
- Describe the signs and symptoms of dactylitis, vaso-occlusive crisis, sepsis, acute chest syndrome, aplastic crisis, splenic sequestration, cerebrovascular accidents and priapism.
- Describe indications for hospital admission, and escalation to intensive care.
- Identify the goals of inpatient therapy, attending to both acute and chronic needs.
- Summarize the roles of members of a comprehensive clinical care team, such as patients, family/caregiver, subspecialty physicians, social worker, pharmacist, physical therapist, discharge planner, psychologist and others.
- Discuss the therapeutic options available for complications of sickle cell disease and describe the rationale for choosing a specific management plan.
- Explain the approach toward acute and chronic pain management.
- Cite reasons for transfer to a referral center in cases requiring pediatric-specific services not available at the local facility.

SKILLS

Pediatric hospitalists should be able to:
- Correctly diagnose sickle cell disease and/or its complications by efficiently performing an accurate history and physical examination, determining if key features of the disease are present.
- Order appropriate laboratory and radiographic testing based on history and physical examination findings.
- Create a comprehensive evaluation and management plan including the use of antimicrobial therapy, intravenous fluid hydration, pain management, transfusion therapy, and initiation of cardiovascular and pulmonary supportive care measures.
- Identify patients with worsening status and respond with appropriate actions.
- Consult subspecialists in a timely manner when appropriate.

ATTITUDES

Pediatric hospitalists should be able to:
- Communicate effectively with patients and the family/caregiver regarding the disease process, expectations of inpatient therapy and transition of care to the outpatient arena.
- Collaborate with subspecialists and the primary care provider and to ensure coordinated longitudinal care for children with sickle cell disease.

SYSTEMS ORGANIZATION AND IMPROVEMENT

In order to improve efficiency and quality within their organizations, pediatric hospitalists should:
- Collaborate with a multidisciplinary team consisting of subspecialty physicians, social workers, pharmacists, physical therapists, discharge planners and psychologists to improve quality of care, increase patient satisfaction and facilitate timely discharge from the acute care setting.
- Identify existing limitations for optimal care within the current hospital setting and work with hospital administration and community partners to develop and sustain appropriate referral systems and coordinated transfers of care.
- Lead, coordinate or participate in the development of coordinated discharge plans and programs in the local community.

SKIN AND SOFT TISSUE INFECTIONS

INTRODUCTION

Skin and soft tissue infections are infections of the skin, subcutaneous tissue and muscle, such as cellulitis or abscess. They do not include infections of the bone, ligaments, cartilage and fibrous tissue. Skin and soft tissue infections are a common cause of hospitalization in children. The most common infectious etiologies of soft tissue infections are streptococcus or staphylococcus species, traditionally treated with Beta-lactam antibiotics. However, infections due to methicillin-resistant staphylococcus aureus, particularly community-acquired methicillin-resistant staphylococcus aureus (CA-MRSA), and other organisms are on the rise. Pediatric hospitalists should be aware of the changing epidemiology of pathogens and resistance patterns to ensure efficient and effective treatment of these infections.

KNOWLEDGE

Pediatric hospitalists should be able to:
- Compare and contrast the key features of the history and physical examination noted in cellulitis versus soft tissue infection.
- Provide indications for hospital admission and determine the appropriate level of care.
- List common bacterial organisms causing skin and soft tissues infections and state how these differ based on age and exposure histories.
- Describe risk factors for infection such as host immunity, dermatoses, environmental exposures and others.
- Discuss the influence of community prevalence of skin pathogens and antimicrobial use on predominant organisms and resistance patterns.

- Review how patient and antibiotic characteristics influence treatment choices.
- List indications for hospitalization.
- Discuss how culture and identification of the organism and susceptibility pattern aids in making treatment decisions, as applicable.
- Compare and contrast emergent versus urgent complications requiring pediatric surgery consultation, such as necrotizing fasciitis and abscesses.
- Explain why early identification and surgical intervention in necrotizing fasciitis can improve outcomes.
- Compare and contrast the utility of various imaging modalities such as plain film, nuclear medicine scan, computed tomography and magnetic resonance imaging and list indications for each.
- Summarize the approach toward evaluation and treatment of patients with recurrent staphylococcal infections, including indications for evaluation for systemic disease, household colonization, and environmental exposures.

SKILLS

Pediatric hospitalists should be able to:
- Demonstrate proficiency in medical interviewing correctly eliciting information such as onset and timing of spread of infection, past history of similar infections, and specific exposures.
- Demonstrate proficiency in conducting a physical examination of skin and soft tissue infections, determining extent and severity of the infection and making proper border demarcations to assist with assessing further spread.
- Order appropriate laboratory and radiographic tests to guide treatment and ensure proper isolation.
- Accurately interpret radiographic studies and engage consultants as appropriate.
- Direct an evidence-based treatment plan including appropriately selected antibiotic therapy attending to the most likely organisms and antibiotic susceptibility patterns.
- Perform careful reassessments daily and as needed, note changes in clinical status, and respond with appropriate actions.
- Adjust antibiotics according to the identification of the organism and/or antibiotic susceptibility pattern and clinical progression/improvement.
- Correctly determine when consultation with a surgeon is indicated.
- Consult appropriate subspecialists early to assist in evaluation and treatment as appropriate.
- Identify patients requiring extended evaluation for underlying anatomic or systemic disease.
- Create a comprehensive discharge plan including home care as appropriate.

ATTITUDES

Pediatric hospitalists should be able to:
- Recognize the importance of consulting with interdisciplinary teams such as pediatric surgeons, radiologists, pharmacists, and the laboratory early in the hospital course to facilitate rapid diagnosis, treatment and discharge.
- Communicate effectively with patients, family/caregiver, primary care provider and subspecialists regarding the reasons for diagnostic testing and treatment choices.
- Educate the family/caregiver on the etiology of the infection, including the importance of hand washing and minimizing environmental exposure in the prevention of infection.
- Display proactive, engaged behavior regarding proper isolation measures to prevent spread of the etiologic agent in the hospital.

SYSTEMS ORGANIZATION AND IMPROVEMENT

In order to improve efficiency and quality within their organizations, pediatric hospitalists should:
- Work with hospital administration and subspecialists to acquire local laboratory testing that is critical for evaluation and management, such as susceptibility testing.
- Incorporate knowledge of outcomes research, changing microbial epidemiology and resistance patterns, cost, and management strategies into patient care.
- Lead, coordinate, or participate in the development and implementation of cost-effective, safe, evidence-based care pathways to standardize the evaluation and management of skin and soft tissue infections.

TOXIC INGESTION

INTRODUCTION

In 2006, the National Data Poison System captured more than 4 million calls to poison control centers in the United States, 2.4 million of which were calls regarding human exposures. More than 50% of reported toxin exposures occur in children under age 6 years. Furthermore, ingestion accounts for 75% of all toxin exposures in younger children. In this age group, toxin ingestion is frequently unintentional and involves non-pharmacologic agents, but therapeutic errors in the administration of pharmacologic agents do occur. In adolescents, toxin ingestion is more often intentional or associated with substance abuse, and carries with it greater morbidity and mortality, particularly when pharmacological agents are involved. Pediatric hospitalists often provide immediate care, coordinate care with subspecialists, or arrange for transfer to another facility when appropriate.

KNOWLEDGE

Pediatric hospitalists should be able to:
- List the pharmacologic and non-pharmacologic agents commonly ingested by pediatric patients and describe how the frequency of each category changes with age.
- Compare and contrast the risk factors and co-morbidities associated with unintentional versus intentional ingestion.
- Describe the signs and symptoms of acute ingestion, including known toxidromes for commonly ingested agents such as salicylates, acetaminophen, narcotics, hallucinogens, stimulants, and others.
- Discuss the risk factors for and presentation of acute and chronic lead poisoning.
- List the laboratory tests that support or refute the diagnosis or assist with the management of common ingestions.
- List the agents detected in locally available blood and urine toxicology screens and describe the benefits and limitations of this testing.
- Explain the indications for and limitations of decontamination therapy, including dermal, ocular, and gastric decontamination methods.
- Identify toxins that have a specific antidote available and explain the indications and limitations of each.
- List local resources that provide information and advice regarding pediatric toxin ingestion management, and recognize there is a single phone number that may be used in the United States to access all regional poison center resources.
- Summarize the indications and goals of hospitalization, attending to acute and chronic medical needs and psychosocial intervention.
- Review the criteria for and process of discharge including psychiatric evaluation, inpatient psychiatric facility transfer, foster care and other elements important for safe discharge.

SKILLS

Pediatric hospitalists should be able to:
- Obtain a focused history, including detailed information about potential exposures, such as the type, amount, and timing of the ingestion.
- Perform a focused physical examination, with attention paid to signs and symptoms that may indicate the ingestion of a particular toxin.
- Efficiently access institutional and local resources to obtain information and advice regarding the diagnosis and management of acute ingestion.
- Identify patients presenting with common toxidromes and efficiently institute appropriate therapy.
- Recognize life-threatening complications such as cardiac dysrhythmias, respiratory depression, or mental status change and institute appropriate therapy in a timely fashion.
- Recognize potential co-morbidities associated with intentional ingestion, such as depression, abuse, or other mental illness.
- Correctly order and interpret basic tests, such as serum chemistries, blood gases, and electrocardiograms, and identify abnormal findings that require additional testing or consultation.
- Develop an appropriate treatment plan based on the presumptive or confirmed agent and provide decontamination or antidote therapy when appropriate.

- Determine the appropriate level of care and duration of observation for a given toxin, recognizing that some agents may have delayed toxic effects.
- Involve subspecialists when appropriate, including social work and/or psychiatric consultation for cases of non-accidental ingestion as appropriate.
- Correctly identify patients who require legal (protective or other) involvement and efficiently access appropriate agencies.

ATTITUDES

Pediatric hospitalists should be able to:
- Counsel the family/caregiver and other professional staff on the possible etiology and outcomes of the ingestion episode.
- Assess the social environment to determine the risk of future exposure and the need for mitigation of risk factors prior to discharge.
- Educate caregivers regarding proactive risk reduction measures, such as the safe and effective storage, use and administration of medications.
- Realize the importance of remaining vigilant regarding changes in recreational drug availability and use as well as safety profile updates on pharmacologic and non-pharmacologic agents.

SYSTEMS ORGANIZATION AND IMPROVEMENT

In order to improve efficiency and quality within their organizations, pediatric hospitalists should:
- Lead, coordinate or participate in the development of systems that integrate hospital, community, and national resources to provide up-to-date and evidence-based information about toxin ingestions and promote timely recognition and treatment of both intentional and unintentional ingestions.
- Lead, coordinate or participate in efforts to educate healthcare providers about the most common ingestions in the pediatric population.
- Lead, coordinate or participate in efforts to educate healthcare providers and the community, regarding ways to mitigate medication errors.

UPPER AIRWAY INFECTIONS

INTRODUCTION

As a group, upper respiratory tract infections in children are responsible for approximately 22 million days of school absence and contribute to work loss due to absence of the family/caregiver caring for ill children. Children under six years of age average six to eight upper respiratory tract infections per year. Although these infections are usually self-limited, they can be associated with airway obstruction and may be life-threatening. Laryngotracheobronchitis (croup) is a common cause of upper airway obstruction in children, affecting up to 6% of children under six years of age. Although less than 5% of children with croup are hospitalized, croup account for 35,000 hospital admissions annually and results in the need for endotracheal intubation for 1-2% of those hospitalized. Other upper airway infections that may lead to airway obstruction include epiglottitis, bacterial tracheitis, severe tonsillitis, and deep neck abscesses. Pediatric hospitalists commonly encounter these patients and are often in the best position to coordinate care across multiple specialties when necessary. Pediatric hospitalists should be able to recognize signs and symptoms of impending or actual airway obstruction, provide immediate care, and arrange for the appropriate subsequent level of care.

KNOWLEDGE

Pediatric hospitalists should be able to:
- Describe the anatomy of the upper respiratory tract and discuss how abnormalities in airflow in different locations may alter clinical presentation.
- Compare and contrast the airway anatomy of neonates, infants, toddlers, preschoolers, school aged children, and adolescents.
- Differentiate between the common infectious etiologies of upper airway obstruction in children of various ages.
- Review alternate diagnoses which may mimic the presentation of acute upper respiratory infection such as allergic reaction, toxic inhalant exposure, and others.

- Describe the signs and symptoms of upper airway obstruction, such as stertor, stridor, "tripod positioning," dysphagia, drooling, trismus and others.
- List the types of radiographic studies available to assess the upper airway (such as plain radiographs, ultrasonography, computed tomography, and magnetic resonance imaging) and discuss the risks, benefits, and indications for each.
- Discuss the indications for nebulized epinephrine, glucocorticoids, antibiotics, and other medications in the treatment of upper respiratory tract infections.
- Compare and contrast the benefits and limitations of various modalities of airway stabilization and respiratory support in patients with varying degrees of upper airway obstruction.
- List the indications for hospital admission, and explain the utility of various monitoring options.
- Discuss the changes in clinical status that indicate need for escalation of care, such as worsening stridor or work of breathing, decreased air entry, cyanosis, altered mental status and others.
- Describe the criteria for management in an intensive care unit or transfer to a tertiary care facility.
- Review the indications for emergent surgical consultation.
- List the criteria for hospital discharge, attending to change in symptoms, oxygenation, hydration, and education.

SKILLS

Pediatric hospitalists should be able to:
- Perform an appropriately focused medical history, attending to symptoms of potential airway obstruction.
- Conduct an appropriate physical examination in children with upper respiratory tract infection, attending to signs and symptoms that may indicate the etiology or severity of the infection.
- Consistently adhere to infection control practices.
- Correctly identify patients with co-morbidities or potential underlying anatomic abnormalities and order appropriate testing and treatment.
- Identify complications of the infection and respond with appropriate actions.
- Perform an evidence-based, cost-effective diagnostic evaluation and treatment plan, avoiding unnecessary testing as appropriate.
- Order appropriate monitoring and correctly interpret monitor data.
- Perform careful reassessments daily and as needed, note changes in clinical status and respond with appropriate actions and escalation of care as appropriate.
- Stabilize the airway and provide appropriate respiratory support for patients with impending or actual airway obstruction or respiratory failure, or arrange for the appropriate personnel to perform the procedure in a timely and safe manner.
- Recognize the indications for and efficiently obtain subspecialty consultation.

ATTITUDES

Pediatric hospitalists should be able to:
- Role model and advocate for strict adherence to infection control practices.
- Communicate effectively with patients and the family/caregiver regarding the diagnosis, management plan, and follow-up needs.
- Collaborate with the primary care provider and subspecialists to ensure a coordinated discharge.

SYSTEMS ORGANIZATION AND IMPROVEMENT

In order to improve efficiency and quality within their organizations, pediatric hospitalists should:
- Lead, coordinate or participate in the development and implementation of cost-effective, safe, evidence-based care within a multidisciplinary team for hospitalized children with upper respiratory tract infections.
- Collaborate with hospital administration and community partners to develop and sustain referral networks between local facilities and tertiary referral centers for hospitalized patients with upper respiratory tract infections.

URINARY TRACT INFECTIONS

INTRODUCTION

Infections of the urinary tract can involve any structure from the kidney to the urethra. Pyelonephritis exists when the infection involves the kidney. Urinary tract infections (UTI) occur in up to 2.8% of all children and 5% of febrile children. They result in 1.1 million office visits (0.7% of total visits) and 13,000 hospitalizations annually. Costs related to only the acute inpatient care of UTI are estimated at $180 million per year alone. The financial impact of subsequent follow-up imaging, treatment, long-term sequelae, and family/caregiver work loss is not well quantitated but is substantial. UTIs may be associated with urologic abnormalities in a significant percentage of young children with pyelonephritis. Pediatric hospitalists frequently encounter children with UTI and must remain current on strategies for diagnosis, treatment and follow-up care for patients with UTIs.

KNOWLEDGE

Pediatric hospitalists should be able to:
- Describe the abnormal anatomic and physiologic aspects of the urogenital system that may predispose children to UTIs at varying ages, such as posterior urethral valves, duplicated system, voiding dysfunction, chronic constipation, and others.
- Describe the range of clinical presentations attending to differences by age.
- Compare and contrast the short and long terms risks of lower versus upper urinary tract infection.
- Define a positive urine culture and discuss how the method for obtaining and efficiency of processing urine influences results of cultures.
- Identify pathogens that cause UTI in both the previously healthy host and those with underlying disease.
- Describe appropriate antibiotic coverage for pathogens of concern with awareness of antibiotic resistance patterns within the local community.
- Discuss the utility of commonly obtained laboratory tests such as urinalysis, urine gram stain, urine culture, blood culture, serum chemistries, and others.
- Review the typical response to therapy, and list common complications of ineffective treatment.
- Summarize current literature regarding treatment and evaluation for underlying abnormalities, including radiography.
- List factors warranting subspecialty consultation or referral.
- Discuss the potential acute and long-term sequelae of treated and untreated UTI.
- Summarize the discharge plan attending to indications for short and long term parenteral and total antimicrobial therapy, repeat evaluations, and subspecialty referral by age.

SKILLS

Pediatric hospitalists should be able to:
- Correctly diagnose UTI by efficiently performing an accurate history and physical examination, determining if key features of the disease are present.
- Identify patients at risk for UTI.
- Order appropriate diagnostic studies for the evaluation of suspected UTI.
- Prescribe appropriate initial antimicrobial and supportive therapy based on history and physical examination.
- Correctly interpret results of diagnostic testing and use results to guide diagnosis and management.
- Correctly identify the need for and efficiently access appropriate consultants and support services needed to provide comprehensive care.
- Identify when discharge criteria are met, and initiate efficient discharge orders and plans.
- Communicate effectively with patients, the family/caregiver and the primary care provider to ensure appropriate post-discharge testing and follow-up.

ATTITUDES

Pediatric hospitalists should be able to:
- Educate the family/caregiver on the expected course of illness, treatment options, and potential sequelae.

- Recognize the importance of communicating with the primary care provider to ensure a safe, efficient, and effective discharge and post-discharge care.
- Collaborate with the healthcare team to ensure coordinated hospital care for children with UTI.

SYSTEMS ORGANIZATION AND IMPROVEMENT

In order to improve efficiency and quality within their organizations, pediatric hospitalists should:
- Collaborate with referring physicians (primary care, emergency medicine, and referring hospital physicians) to develop and sustain appropriate referral networks for evaluation, admission, or transfer of children with UTI.
- Collaborate with subspecialists to ensure consistent, timely, and up-to-date evaluation and care in the inpatient setting.
- Lead, coordinate or participate in the development and implementation of cost-effective, safe, evidence-based care pathways to standardize the evaluation and management of hospitalized children with UTI.

Pediatric Hospital Medicine Core Competencies

Section Two: Core Skills

BLADDER CATHETERIZATION/SUPRAPUBIC BLADDER TAP

INTRODUCTION

Bladder catheterization is a common procedure, typically used to collect a sterile urine sample for analysis and culture when urinary tract infection is suspected. Bladder catheterization is also used to relieve urinary retention or obstruction, particularly in cases of anatomic abnormalities or neurogenic bladder, or to monitor urine output and fluid status. Pediatric hospitalists frequently encounter patients requiring bladder catheterization and should be adept at performing this procedure in infants, children, and adolescents.

KNOWLEDGE

Pediatric hospitalists should be able to:

- List the indications and contraindications for bladder catheterization.
- Describe how the method used to collect a urine specimen can affect interpretation of urine culture results, and explain why bladder catheterization or suprapubic tap are the preferred methods of collection in infants and children that cannot reliably produce a voided specimen.
- Review the basic anatomy of the male and female genitourinary tract.
- Review the steps in performing bladder catheterization for both male and female patients, attending to aspects such as patient identification, sterile technique, positioning, equipment needs, and specimen handling.
- Discuss the indications for analgesia, sedation, or anxiolysis and describe the medications that may be used for each.
- Describe the risks and complications associated with bladder catheterization, such as localized trauma, creation of a false passage, and potential stricture formation.
- List the indications for consultation with a urologist with regard to bladder catheterization, including known genitourinary tract abnormality, recent genitourinary surgery, or urethral trauma
- Compare and contrast the effects of using various methods to collect a urine specimen, including interpretation of the culture and urinalysis and patient risk,
- Define a UTI as obtained by various methods such as catheterization, clean catch, clean bag, and suprapubic tap.
- Discuss the importance of appropriate specimen handling and the effect on culture results.

SKILLS

Pediatric hospitalists should be able to:

- Perform a pre-procedural evaluation to determine risks and benefits of bladder catheterization.
- Demonstrate proficiency in performance of bladder catheterization on infants, children, and adolescents.
- Consider the level of pain and anxiety provoked by the procedure and provide appropriate pharmacologic or non-pharmacologic interventions when indicated.
- Correctly identify the need for and efficiently offer education to healthcare providers on proper techniques for holding and calming patients before, during, and after bladder catheterization.
- Consistently adhere to infection control practices.
- Identify complications and respond with appropriate actions.
- Identify the need for and efficiently access appropriate consultants and support services for assistance with analgesia, sedation, anxiolysis, and performance of a bladder catheterization.

ATTITUDES

Hospital physicians should be able to:

- Recognize the importance of obtaining a sterile urine specimen in order to correctly diagnose urinary tract infection.
- Communicate effectively with patients and the family/caregiver regarding the indications for, risks, benefits, and steps of bladder catheterization.
- Role model and advocate for strict adherence to infection control practices

SYSTEMS ORGANIZATION AND IMPROVEMENT

In order to improve efficiency and quality within their organizations, pediatric hospitalists should:
- Lead, coordinate or participate in the development and implementation of cost-effective, safe, evidence-based procedures and policies for performance of bladder catheterization in children.
- Lead, coordinate or participate in the development and implementation of educational initiatives designed to teach the proper technique for bladder catheterization to learners and other healthcare providers.

ELECTROCARDIOGRAM INTERPRETATION

INTRODUCTION

Cardiorespiratory monitoring is used commonly during hospitalization, and electrocardiograms (ECGs) are often obtained to screen for or diagnose cardiac pathology. Cardiac arrhythmias in the hospital setting can be of clinical significance and may be life-threatening. Early recognition of a clinically significant arrhythmia will result in rapid implementation of appropriate and life-saving interventions. Pediatric hospitalists are often in the best position to recognize, diagnose, and provide the initial treatment for cardiac arrhythmias and other cardiac problems. Pediatric hospitalists should be skilled at obtaining and interpreting ECGs.

KNOWLEDGE

Pediatric hospitalists should be able to:
- Describe the normal electrical cardiac cycle and the corresponding wave forms on an ECG tracing.
- Review the steps in performing an ECG, attending to lead placement and other technical aspects of the procedure.
- Summarize a general approach to the interpretation of pediatric ECGs, attending to evaluation of heart rate, rhythm, QRS axis, wave form durations and intervals, and chamber hypertrophy.
- Compare and contrast the features of the newborn ECG to those of older children and adults.
- Describe the common ECG changes associated with specific electrolyte disturbances.
- List the medications associated with potentially serious arrhythmias (e.g. cisapride and prolonged QT syndrome).
- Describe the appropriate treatment for specific cardiac arrhythmias (e.g. medications, electrical cardioversion, or defibrillation).
- List the ECG findings that should prompt consultation with a cardiologist, including life-threatening or unstable cardiac arrhythmia.

SKILLS

Pediatric hospitalists should be able to:
- Obtain an ECG using the standard number and placement of leads, recording speed, and sensitivity.
- Differentiate between a normal sinus rhythm and other rhythms by evaluating the presence and relationship of the P wave to the QRS complex.
- Determine the heart rate, considering both the atrial and ventricular rates if different.
- Determine the PR and QT intervals, P and QRS durations, and QRS axis.
- Calculate the corrected QT interval (QTc) for the evaluation of prolonged QT syndrome.
- Use the calculated intervals, durations, and amplitudes to evaluate for chamber hypertrophy and to screen for ischemia.
- Recognize patterns that are pathognomonic for certain diagnoses (e.g., delta waves in Wolff-Parkinson-White syndrome).
- Correctly identify abnormal cardiac rhythms and respond with appropriate actions and interventions, including medications, electrical cardioversion, and defibrillation.
- Order appropriate monitoring and correctly interpret monitor data.
- Consult a pediatric cardiologist when indicated.

ATTITUDES

Pediatric hospitalists should be able to:
- Assume responsibility for the need to obtain an ECG and provide an accurate interpretation.
- Communicate effectively with patients, the family/caregivers and other healthcare providers regarding the need to obtain an ECG, findings, and care plan.
- Collaborate with the primary care provider and subspecialists to ensure coordinated longitudinal care for children with cardiac pathology.

SYSTEMS ORGANIZATION AND IMPROVEMENT

In order to improve efficiency and quality within their organizations, Pediatric Hospitalists should:
- Lead, coordinate, or participate in the development and implementation of cost-effective and evidence-based policies regarding the indications for obtaining an ECG.
- Work with pediatric cardiologists, hospital staff, and others to ensure timely, reliable and accurate pediatric ECG interpretation.
- Lead, coordinate, or participate in efforts directed at educating healthcare providers about risk factors for cardiac arrhythmia, early identification of abnormal rhythms, and implementation of appropriate resuscitative efforts.

FEEDING TUBES

INTRODUCTION

Feeding tubes are commonly used to deliver enteral nutrition and medications to pediatric inpatients. Commonly used tubes are nasogastric (NG), nasojejunal (NJ), gastric (G), gastrojejunal (GJ), or jejunal (J). They may be used instead of or in addition to oral feedings. Feeding tubes may deliver nutrition and medications into the stomach or past the pylorus. While different types of feeding tubes may be placed by a variety of practitioners - nurses, radiologists, medical physicians, or surgeons - it is critical for pediatric hospitalists to understand the uses, limitations, and complications of various types of feeding tubes.

KNOWLEDGE

Pediatric hospitalists should be able to:
- Describe basic gastrointestinal anatomy and physiology, and relate this to commonly used feeding tubes.
- Compare and contrast the indications, uses, and limitations of various types of feeding tubes, including NG, NJ, G, GJ, and J tubes.
- Discuss the benefits of short term enteral feeding compared to intravenous fluid or parenteral nutrition use.
- Describe the correct procedure to replace each type of feeding tube and potential complications to be avoided.
- Review commonly encountered short and long term complications of feeding tubes, such as nasal irritation, granulation tissue, cellulitis, extrusion, obstruction, and others.
- Compare and contrast risks and benefits of percutaneous endoscopic gastrostomy (PEG) versus surgical gastrostomy.
- List the indications, risks, benefits, and alternatives for surgical gastrostomy with Nissen fundoplication.
- Discuss the factors to consider when determining the optimal type of feeding tube for children with neurologic impairment, such as risk of aspiration pneumonia, social aspects of maintaining oral stimulation, complications of Nissen fundoplication, and others.
- Compare and contrast the short and long term risks and benefits of gastrostomy with Nissen fundoplication versus placement of GJ tubes in patients with neurologic impairment.
- Discuss the roles of primary care provider, home care, subspecialists, and the family/caregiver in the home management of feeding tubes.

SKILLS

Pediatric hospitalists should be able to:
- Correctly institute short term NG feeding in appropriate patients.
- Appropriately prescribe NG or NJ feeding, including correct starting and increasing volumes and enteral formula choice.

- Correctly identify and refer appropriate patients for a G tube, GJ tube, or J tube placement.
- Effectively and clearly articulate the risks and benefits of combining Nissen Fundoplication with G tube placement vs. GJ tube placement to the family/caregiver.
- Accurately diagnose and treat dermatological problems associated with feeding tubes.
- Accurately diagnose and initiate treatment for common complications (obstruction, extrusion, leakage) associated with feeding tubes, in collaboration with appropriate subspecialists.
- Order appropriate radiological studies to assess feeding tube dysfunction.
- Demonstrate basic proficiency in interpretation of radiographic studies commonly performed to assess correct tube placement.
- Correctly identify the need for and efficiently access appropriate consultants.

ATTITUDES

Pediatric hospitalists should be able to:
- Work collaboratively with patients, family/caregiver, hospital staff, subspecialists and the primary care provider in making decisions regarding feeding tubes.
- Elicit and allay concerns of patients and the family/caregiver regarding the cosmetic appearance of tubes or impact on oral feeding.
- Educate patients and the family/caregiver about the use and care of feeding tubes prior to discharge home.
- Recognize the key role that home health care plays in the discharge planning and long term care of children with feeding tubes.

SYSTEMS ORGANIZATION AND IMPROVEMENT

In order to improve efficiency and quality within their organizations, pediatric hospitalists should:
- Lead, coordinate or participate in the development and implementation of cost-effective, safe, evidence-based care pathways to standardize the evaluation and management of feeding tubes for children.
- Collaborate with hospital administration and community partners to develop and sustain local systems that organize and consolidate the feeding tube supplies and services for children in an identifiable, easily accessible location.
- Lead, coordinate or participate in efforts to develop strategies to minimize institutional complication rates from feeding tube placement and use.
- Lead, coordinate or participate in multidisciplinary efforts to develop an education and hospital discharge protocol to ensure that patients with feeding tubes are safely transitioned to the outpatient setting.

FLUID AND ELECTROLYTE MANAGEMENT

INTRODUCTION

Many infants and children are hospitalized in the United States each year for fluid and electrolyte disorders. Dehydration from gastroenteritis alone accounts for more than 200,000 pediatric hospitalizations each year. An understanding of pediatric fluid therapy is one of the most important advances of pediatric medicine and a cornerstone of current inpatient pediatric practice. Although the majority of previously healthy hospitalized children can compensate for errors in calculations of fluid therapy, mistakes, even in healthy children admitted for minor illnesses, can have devastating outcomes. Patients with underlying disease processes are at even greater risk for adverse outcomes if fluids and electrolytes are not meticulously managed. Pediatric hospitalists should be experts at managing frequently encountered fluid and electrolyte abnormalities.

KNOWLEDGE

Pediatric hospitalists should be able to:
- Discuss the physiology of fluid and electrolyte homeostasis and the changes that occur with growth and development.
- Discuss how maintenance fluid calculations are based upon water and electrolyte homeostasis using various methods such as the body surface area or Holliday Segar methods. Describe the methods used for calculation of excessive fluid losses due to causes such as diarrhea, increased ostomy output, burns, and vomiting; identify the best fluid replacement type for each.

- Describe common errors in clinical estimations of dehydration and fluid and electrolyte requirements.
- Explain the rationale, indications and contraindications for oral rehydration, including the correct glucose and electrolyte composition and technique for administration.
- Discuss the benefits of and barriers to use of nasogastric tubes for administering enteral fluids.
- Discuss the options and indications for different methods of parenteral fluid administration, including intravenous, intraosseous, and subcutaneous.
- Review the indications for administering a parenteral fluid bolus for resuscitation and explain the rationale for the use of isotonic fluids for rehydration.
- Discuss the benefits and risks of repeated lab testing and intravenous access placement, including cost, pain, effect on clinical management, family/caregiver perceptions, staff time, and others.
- Compare and contrast true hyponatremia with pseudohyponatremia and give examples of conditions in which these exist.
- List differential diagnoses for hyponatremia and hypernatremia.
- Summarize the management of hypo- and hypernatremia, attending to duration of corrective therapy and potential complications during correction.
- Distinguish between hyperkalemia and pseudohyperkalemia and give examples of the conditions in which these exist.
- List differential diagnoses for hypokalemia and hyperkalemia.
- Distinguish hypocalcemia from pseudohypocalcemia and give examples of the conditions in which these exist.
- Discuss the interaction of fluid and electrolytes with acid/base balance.
- Describe common acid/base disturbances that accompany the most frequently encountered causes of fluid deficit and give examples of exacerbating issues such as underlying co-morbidity and use of over-the-counter medications.

SKILLS

Pediatric hospitalists should be able to:
- Accurately calculate maintenance fluid and electrolyte requirements for hospitalized infants and children.
- Promptly adjust maintenance fluids for increased insensible losses and ongoing fluid and electrolyte needs.
- Estimate the degree of dehydration for children of various ages based upon clinical symptoms and signs.
- Recognize common presenting signs and symptoms in infants and children that are associated with an excess or deficit of each common electrolyte and glucose.
- Correctly estimate osmolar disturbance by interpreting electrolyte, glucose and blood urea nitrogen results.
- Calculate and administer an isotonic fluid bolus correctly when indicated.
- Obtain intravenous or intraosseous access in moderate to severely dehydrated patients.
- Assess the success of fluid resuscitation by interpreting clinical change and laboratory values.
- Calculate and administer maintenance and deficit fluid replacement for isotonic, hypertonic, and hypotonic dehydration.
- Interpret urine and serum electrolytes and osmolality, as well as fluid status (hypo, hyper or isovolemic), to determine the etiology for hyponatremia or hypernatremia.
- Correct hyponatremia using appropriate replacement or restriction of fluids, sodium chloride, and medications depending upon the diagnosis.
- Correct hypernatremia using an appropriate electrolyte composition and rate of fluid replacement, as well as medications depending upon the diagnosis.
- Correct hypoglycemia using an appropriate replacement solution.
- Interpret EKG findings in the context of specific electrolyte abnormalities.
- Safely prescribe electrolyte replacement therapy and institute proper monitoring for arrhythmias.
- Correct symptomatic hyperkalemia using a combination of therapies to stabilize cardiac conduction, redistribute potassium to the intracellular space and remove it from the body.

ATTITUDES

Pediatric hospitalists should be able to:
- Consult pediatric subspecialists appropriately to expedite the diagnosis and management of serious electrolyte disorders.

- Recognize the benefits of oral rehydration and advocate for its use when indicated and clinically appropriate.
- Coordinate subspecialty and primary care follow up for patients with persistent disturbances at discharge as appropriate.
- Consider cost-effectiveness, pain, and patient safety when creating plans for the treatment of fluid deficits.

SYSTEMS ORGANIZATION AND IMPROVEMENT

In order to improve efficiency and quality within their organizations, pediatric hospitalists should:
- Lead, coordinate or participate in plans to develop institutional policies to safely monitor and administer fluids and electrolytes.
- Work collaboratively with others such as surgeons, intensivists, and advanced practice nurses to establish venous access when needed.
- Lead, coordinate or participate in developing guidelines for the treatment of fluid and electrolyte abnormalities in the hospital and community.

INTRAVENOUS ACCESS AND PHLEBOTOMY

INTRODUCTION

Intravenous (IV) access is the most common procedure performed on a pediatric inpatient unit. IV access may be used for immediate fluid resuscitation, parenteral medication or nutrition delivery, or be placed in anticipation of need for emergent access for medications for patients at risk for acute deterioration such as possible seizure or respiratory compromise. Pediatric hospitalists should be adept at obtaining peripheral IV access in all pediatric patients, and IV or intraosseous (IO) access in critically ill patients. Although not a requirement, many pediatric hospitalists may also obtain skills in the placement of other forms of intravenous access, including central venous catheters and percutaneously inserted central catheters (PICC). Pediatric hospitalists are also often in the best position to obtain venous and arterial blood samples from pediatric patients. Adequate discussion with patients and family/caregiver, and appropriate use of topical anesthesia, anxiolysis, or minimal sedation can create the environment needed for a successful procedure.

KNOWLEDGE

Pediatric hospitalists should be able to:
- List the indications for intravenous access such as rehydration or resuscitation, parenteral administration of medications and others.
- Describe common complications of both peripheral and central IV access, including infiltration, bleeding, infection, and thrombosis.
- Compare and contrast the risks and benefits of using peripheral versus central sites for IV access as well as line type, attending to indications and complications for each.
- List the indications for arterial blood sampling.
- Review the proper method for obtaining venous and arterial blood samples.
- Discuss how anatomic location of veins and arteries influences the catheterization technique.
- Describe common complications from venous and arterial blood sampling.
- Discuss how factors such as age, disease process, and anatomy influence the choice of IV site.
- Summarize current literature and national best practices regarding avoidance of catheter-related bloodstream infections.
- Review the options for pain and sedation management, attending to medication and non-medication interventions by age and developmental stage.
- Review methods which can help minimize the number of IV attempts and discuss common complications from IV attempts.
- State why use of certain existing and potential venous sites (such as hemodialysis catheters, limb with neurovascular compromise, and others) is contraindicated.
- State the relative contraindications to certain IV access sites such as jugular veins with a neighboring ventriculoperitoneal shunt, fracture in limb and others.
- State the indications and contraindications for IO access.

- Describe the indications, risks, benefits, and alternatives for PICC placement attending to prolonged medication and/or nutrition needs.
- Review the common radiographic modalities used to assess proper line placement and function.
- Review the indications for subspecialty consultation for IV access or blood sampling, and list commonly accessed subspecialty services, attending to local context.

SKILLS

Pediatric hospitalists should be able to:
- Perform a pre-procedural evaluation to determine risks and benefits of IV placement.
- Correctly assess the need for and order appropriate pain and sedation medication and non-medication interventions.
- Obtain IV access on children of all ages.
- Demonstrate proficiency in performing venous and arterial blood sampling (phlebotomy) with and without IV access.
- Correctly identify the need for and efficiently offer education to healthcare providers on proper techniques for holding and calming patients before, during, and after access attempts.
- Consistently adhere to infection control practices.
- Demonstrate proficiency with intraosseous needle placement during emergency situations, and successfully insert the IO needle into a simulator in mock code situations at least once per year.
- Identify barriers to efficient, effective IV access and engage subspecialists to assist as appropriate.
- Demonstrate proficiency in performing or efficiently accessing appropriate consultants to perform central venous access and PICC lines.
- Identify common complications of IVs and blood sampling and respond with appropriate actions.
- Demonstrate proficiency in performing or efficiently accessing appropriate consultants to perform basic repairs on central venous lines and PICC lines.

ATTITUDES

Pediatric hospitalists should be able to:
- Work collaboratively with hospital staff and subspecialists to ensure coordinated planning and performance of IV access.
- Communicate effectively with patients and the family/caregiver regarding the indications for, risks, benefits, and steps of the procedure.
- Role model and advocate for strict adherence to infection control practices.

SYSTEMS ORGANIZATION AND IMPROVEMENT

In order to improve efficiency and quality within their organizations, pediatric hospitalists should:
- Lead, coordinate or participate in the development and implementation of cost-effective, safe, evidence-based procedures and policies for IV access following national guidelines for infection control.
- Work with hospital administration, hospital staff and others to develop and implement standardized documentation tools for venous access procedures.
- Lead, coordinate or participate in the development and implementation of a system for review of the efficacy, efficiency and outcomes of intravenous access procedures.
- Lead, coordinate or participate in the development and implementation of a system for review of family/caregiver and healthcare provider satisfaction into procedural strategies.

LUMBAR PUNCTURE

INTRODUCTION

Lumbar puncture is a common typically performed procedure to confirm clinical suspicion of meningitis. Other common indications include the evaluation and diagnosis of pseudotumor cerebri, complex migraine headaches, altered mental status, subarachnoid hemorrhage, neurologic deterioration, and demyelinating diseases such as Guillan Barré. A lumbar puncture or "spinal tap" often elicits great concern from both patients and the family/caregiver due to a misunderstanding of risk to the spinal cord. Adequate discussion with patients and the family/caregiver, and appropriate use of topical anesthesia, anxiolysis, or sedation can create the environment needed for a successful procedure. Pediatric hospitalists frequently encounter patients requiring lumbar puncture and should be adept at performing lumbar puncture in all appropriately selected pediatric patients.

KNOWLEDGE

Pediatric hospitalists should be able to:
- List the indications for lumbar puncture, such as confirmation of pleocytosis, aiding initial antimicrobial selection, therapeutic removal of fluid, assessment of response to treatment, performance of neurometabolic studies, and others.
- Review the basic anatomy of the spine and spinal column.
- List the indications for obtaining an imaging study of the brain or spinal cord prior to performing a lumbar puncture.
- Describe the relative contraindications to lumbar puncture such as pre-existing ventriculoperitoneal shunt or previous spinal surgeries and discuss the options for safely obtaining cerebrospinal fluid in these patients
- List the absolute contraindications to lumbar puncture, such as increased intracranial pressure, unstable cardiorespiratory status, unstable coagulopathies, and others.
- Describe the risks and complications of lumbar puncture attending to infection, bleeding, nerve injury, pain, post-procedure headache, and others.
- Summarize factors that may increase risk for complications such as age, disease process, and anatomy.
- Review the steps in performing a lumbar puncture, attending to aspects such as infection control, patient identification, positioning options, monitoring, family/caregiver presence and others.
- Discuss the roles of each member of the healthcare team, attending to proper level of monitoring to maximize safety, timeout, documentation, specimen labeling and transport to the laboratory, and communication with patients and the family/caregiver.

SKILLS

Pediatric hospitalists should be able to:
- Perform a pre-procedural evaluation to determine risks and benefits of lumbar puncture.
- Correctly obtain informed consent from the family/caregiver.
- Correctly order and ensure proper performance of procedural sedation if indicated, including assurance of adequate number of staff present for both the lumbar puncture and the sedation.
- Demonstrate proficiency in performance of lumbar puncture on infants, children, and adolescents.
- Correctly identify the need for and efficiently offer education to healthcare providers on proper techniques for holding and calming patients before, during, and after lumbar puncture attempts.
- Consistently adhere to infection control practices.
- Order appropriate monitoring and correctly interpret monitor data.
- Identify complications and respond with appropriate actions.
- Accurately use the pressure manometer as appropriate.
- Correctly identify the need for and efficiently access appropriate consultants and support services for assistance with pain management, sedation, and performance of a lumbar puncture.

ATTITUDES

Pediatric hospitalists should be able to:
- Work collaboratively with hospital staff and subspecialists to ensure coordinated planning and performance of lumbar punctures.
- Communicate effectively with patients and the family/caregiver regarding the indications for, risks, benefits, and steps of the procedure.
- Role model and advocate for strict adherence to infection control practices.

SYSTEMS ORGANIZATION AND IMPROVEMENT

In order to improve efficiency and quality within their organizations, pediatric hospitalists should:
- Lead, coordinate or participate in the development and implementation of cost-effective, safe, evidence-based procedures and policies for performance of lumbar punctures for children.
- Work with hospital administration, hospital staff and others to develop and implement standardized documentation tools for the procedure.
- Lead, coordinate or participate in the development and implementation of a system for review of family/ caregiver and healthcare provider satisfaction into procedural strategies.

NON-INVASIVE MONITORING

INTRODUCTION

Collection and monitoring of objective data such as vital signs and pulse oximetry measurements are essential components of care for hospitalized children. Combined with clinical assessments, these data are critical when making therapeutic or diagnostic decisions. A complete understanding of non-invasive monitoring techniques is necessary to accurately interpret the data generated. Pediatric hospitalists regularly incorporate this data into their clinical practice and, especially when overseeing procedural sedation or emergent clinical situations, may be responsible for implementing or supervising the appropriate type and level of monitoring.

KNOWLEDGE

Pediatric hospitalists should be able to:
- List the different types of non-invasive monitoring techniques and devices that are available and describe the indications for each.
- Compare and contrast the types and level of monitoring generally available on the inpatient ward compared to the intensive care unit or other care settings.
- Describe the proper procedures for common non-invasive monitoring techniques, including vital sign measurement, cardiopulmonary monitoring, pulse oximetry, and capnography.
- List the limitations or complications associated with common non-invasive monitoring techniques, such as inadequate wave form for pulse oximetry.
- Discuss the importance of accurate and timely interpretation of information generated by monitoring devices, as well as the importance of an immediate response when abnormal data is noted.

SKILLS

Pediatric hospitalists should be able to:
- Determine the type and level of monitoring needed based on the clinical situation and medical complexity of the patient.
- Identify the need for a higher or lower level of monitoring as changes in the clinical status occur and transfer the patient to the appropriate inpatient setting.
- Ensure proper placement of monitoring equipment (e.g., placement of monitor leads) and execution of proper technique (e.g., use of correct size blood pressure cuff) in order to obtain accurate data.
- Correctly interpret monitoring data and respond with appropriate actions.

ATTITUDES

Pediatric hospitalists should be able to:
- Assume responsibility for ordering the appropriate monitoring and interpreting monitoring data.
- Collaborate with nurses, subspecialists, and other healthcare providers to determine the appropriate level of monitoring and the corresponding care setting, especially when clinical changes occur.
- Communicate effectively with patients and the family/caregiver regarding the need for non-invasive monitoring, the findings, and the care plan.

SYSTEMS ORGANIZATION AND IMPROVEMENT

In order to improve efficiency and quality within their organizations, pediatric hospitalists should:
- Lead, coordinate, or participate in the development and implementation of cost-effective, safe, evidence-based procedures and policies related to non-invasive monitoring.
- Work with hospital administration, biomedical engineering, and others to obtain high quality and reliable monitoring equipment.
- Lead, coordinate, or participate in the development of continuing education programs focused on non-invasive monitoring and the interpretation of related data.
- Lead, coordinate or participate in the development and implementation of a system for review of family/caregiver and healthcare provider satisfaction into monitoring strategies.

NUTRITION

INTRODUCTION

Optimal nutrition in the hospital setting has been shown to improve outcomes in adult patients, and there is a growing body of evidence that the same is true for pediatric patients. Malnutrition refers to any disorder of nutritional status resulting from a deficiency or excess of nutrient intake, imbalance of essential nutrients, or impaired nutrient metabolism. Malnutrition occurs in up to half of hospitalized children in the United States, but varies considerably by age and disease state. An understanding of the fundamental nutritional requirements of pediatric patients is essential to providing optimal care for hospitalized children. Pediatric hospitalists should be experts in making objective nutritional assessments and managing frequently encountered nutritional problems. Pediatric hospitalists should lead, coordinate, or participate in multidisciplinary efforts to screen for malnutrition and improve the nutritional status of hospitalized pediatric patients.

KNOWLEDGE

Pediatric hospitalists should be able to:
- Describe the normal growth patterns for children at various ages and the potential effect of malnutrition on growth.
- List the anthropometric measurements commonly used to assess acute and chronic nutritional status.
- Describe the basic nutritional requirements for hospitalized pediatric patients, based on gestational age, chronologic age, weight, activity level, and other characteristics.
- Compare and contrast the composition of human milk versus commonly used commercial formulas, and explain why human milk is superior nutrition for infants.
- Describe the differences in composition of commonly used commercial formulas, as well as protein hydrosylate and other special formulas, and list the clinical indications for each type of formula.
- Compare and contrast the benefits and costs of blended foods versus commonly used enteral formulas as complete nutritional sources for children receiving gastric, duodenal, or jejunal tube feedings.
- List the indications for specific vitamin and mineral supplementation, including exclusive breastfeeding, chronic anti-epileptic therapy, food allergies resulting in extreme dietary restrictions, and others.
- List the factors that place hospitalized pediatric patients at risk for poor nutrition.
- Compare and contrast marasmus and kwashiorkor.
- Define the term protein-energy malnutrition.
- List the signs and symptoms of common vitamin and mineral deficiencies.
- List the indications and contraindications for both enteral and parenteral nutrition, and describe the complications associated with each type of supplemental nutrition.
- Discuss the monitoring needs for pediatric patients on chronic enteral or parenteral nutrition attending to electrolyte and mineral disturbances, growth, and other parameters.
- Describe the refeeding syndrome and list the risk factors associated with its development.
- Explain the importance of nutrition screening, as well as the indications for consultation with a nutritionist, gastroenterologist, or other subspecialist.

SKILLS

Pediatric hospitalists should be able to:
- Use anthropometric data to determine the presence, degree, and chronicity of malnutrition.
- Conduct a focused history and physical examination, attending to details that may indicate a particular nutrient, vitamin, or mineral deficiency.
- Conduct a directed laboratory evaluation to obtain information about nutritional status and vitamin or mineral deficiencies, as indicated.
- Calculate the basic caloric, protein, fat, and fluid requirements for hospitalized pediatric patients, for both daily needs and catch up growth.
- Provide lactation support to all mothers, especially those who are experiencing difficulty with initiating or maintaining breastfeeding or milk supply or those who have a complication from breastfeeding, including plugged ducts or mastitis.
- Choose an appropriate formula, delivery device, and method of administration when enteral nutrition is required.
- Initiate and advance parenteral nutrition using the appropriate initial composition of parenteral nutrition solution, delivery device, and method of administration when parenteral nutrition is required.
- Appropriately monitor laboratory values to ensure the efficacy of supplemental nutrition support and to screen for complications.
- Recognize and treat complications of both enteral and parenteral nutrition, such as metabolic derangements, infection, and delivery device malfunction.
- Recognize and treat the refeeding syndrome.
- Consult a nutritionist, gastroenterologist, or other subspecialists when indicated.

ATTITUDES

Pediatric hospitalists should be able to:
- Recognize the importance of screening for malnutrition and optimizing nutritional status for hospitalized pediatric patients.
- Communicate effectively with patients, the family/caregiver, and healthcare providers regarding findings and care plans.
- Collaborate with a nutritionist or subspecialists to devise and implement a nutrition care plan.
- Collaborate with the primary care provider and subspecialists to ensure coordinated, longitudinal care for children requiring specialized nutrition support.
- Arrange for an effective and safe transition of care from the inpatient to outpatient providers, preserving the multidisciplinary nature of the nutrition care team when appropriate.

SYSTEMS ORGANIZATION AND IMPROVEMENT

In order to improve efficiency and quality within their organizations, pediatric hospitalists should:
- Lead, coordinate, or participate in efforts to develop systems that support the initiation and maintenance of breastfeeding for infants
- Work with hospital administration, hospital staff, subspecialists, and other services/consultants to promote prompt nutritional screening for all hospitalized patients and multidisciplinary team care to address nutritional problems when indicated.
- Lead, coordinate or participate in the development and implementation of cost-effective, evidence-based care pathways to standardize the evaluation and management for hospitalized children with nutritional needs

OXYGEN DELIVERY AND AIRWAY MANAGEMENT

INTRODUCTION

Respiratory distress and respiratory failure account for a significant number of pediatric emergencies in the acute care and inpatient settings. In these situations, early identification and treatment of respiratory compromise is critical. Appropriate airway management and oxygen delivery will result in reduced morbidity and mortality. Pediatric hospitalists frequently encounter children with respiratory compromise and are often in the best position to provide immediate, life-saving interventions.

KNOWLEDGE

Pediatric hospitalists should be able to:

- Review the basic anatomy of the upper respiratory tract and describe the anatomic differences between infants, children, and adolescents.
- Describe the various forms of monitoring related to assessment of oxygenation and ventilation, including cardiorespiratory monitors, pulse oximetry, capnography, and blood gas sampling.
- List the crucial items to have available at the bedside or in an emergency supply cart in the event of respiratory compromise, including suction, oxygen, oxygen delivery systems, pediatric sizes of advanced airway equipment, and resuscitation medications.
- Summarize the steps involved in assessing and securing a patient's airway, including proper airway positioning, suctioning, selection and use of the appropriate airway equipment, and the use of adjunctive medications.
- Describe the indications for and uses of different types of airway equipment, including oropharyngeal, nasopharyngeal, laryngeal mask, and tracheal airways.
- Compare and contrast low flow and high flow oxygen delivery systems, and give examples of each.
- Describe the mechanism of action of heliox and inhaled nitric oxide and list the indications for their use.
- List factors that may complicate airway management, including anatomic abnormalities of the face and oropharynx, neurologic impairment, and trauma.
- List the indications for consultation with an otorhinolaryngologist, anesthesiologist, or other subspecialist with regard to airway management.

SKILLS

Pediatric hospitalists should be able to:

- Anticipate the need for airway management or oxygen delivery and ensure that all appropriate equipment is readily available.
- Perform frequent clinical assessments and recognize when patients need supplemental oxygen or airway management.
- Correctly position the pediatric airway using head tilt and jaw thrust maneuvers.
- Use suction equipment to clear the airway when necessary.
- Select and use the appropriate method for oxygen delivery when indicated.
- Select the appropriate airway device and establish a secure airway when indicated.
- For patients with established tracheostomy tubes, respond with appropriate actions when the tube becomes obstructed or dislodged.
- Select appropriate monitoring and correctly interpret monitor data.
- Correctly identify the needs for and efficiently access appropriate consultants to ensure proper airway management.
- Implement an appropriate respiratory care plan for ongoing patient management, collaborating with nursing staff, respiratory therapy, subspecialists, and other healthcare providers as indicated.

ATTITUDES

Pediatric hospitalists should be able to:

- Assume responsibility for airway management and oxygen delivery.
- Recognize the importance of maintaining skills in airway management and oxygen delivery and participate in relevant continuing education activities.
- Communicate effectively with patients and the family/caregiver regarding the need for airway management or oxygen delivery and the care plan.

SYSTEMS ORGANIZATION AND IMPROVEMENT

In order to improve efficiency and quality within their organizations, pediatric hospitalists should:

- Lead, coordinate, or participate in the development of hospital systems designed to detect patients with respiratory compromise early and provide an appropriate, rapid response.

- Lead, coordinate, or participate in educational initiatives for nurses, physicians, and other healthcare providers related to pediatric advanced life support.
- Work with hospital administration to ensure emergency code carts are pediatric-specific and contain adequate, appropriate equipment.
- Lead, coordinate, or participate in peer review or relevant case conferences with subspecialists and other healthcare providers to identify individual areas or systems issues in need if improvement.

PAIN MANAGEMENT

INTRODUCTION

Acute pain (pain) is a common complaint in the pediatric inpatient setting and is most often associated with exacerbations of chronic diseases, trauma, burns or surgical and diagnostic procedures. Children with acute pain may also have chronic pain due to an underlying illness or previous injury. Chronic pain complicates effective control of acute pain and may be associated with neuropsychological changes that impact pain perception. Despite advances in understanding of the pathophysiology and management of pain in children, several barriers to effective pain management exist, such as fear of harmful side effects and drug dependency. Pediatric hospitalists should enhance pain management services through the direct provision of effective care, and are often in the best position to lead development of a systematic approach to pain management in institutions and communities.

KNOWLEDGE

Pediatric hospitalists should be able to:
- Describe the pathophysiology and multidimensional aspects of pain in children of various ages.
- Explain how pain, anxiety, and fear interrelate and discuss strategies for addressing each.
- List the indications and contraindications for the main classes of drugs used for pain management, such as opioids, non-steroidal anti-inflammatory drugs, and topical and local anesthetics.
- Discuss the pharmacology of medications commonly used for analgesia, including route of administration, dosing range, and expected side effects.
- Discuss the pharmacology of medications used for anxiolysis, including route of administration, dosing range, and expected side effects.
- Describe the effects of age, anatomy, and disease process on the pharmacology of medications used for analgesia and anxiolysis.
- Compare and contrast the risks and benefits of various modalities of drug delivery attending to drug delivery, side effects, and invasiveness and safety of delivery methods/devices.
- List appropriate monitoring techniques for patients receiving analgesics, anxiolytics, and other associated medications.
- Describe the pharmacology of and indications for reversal agents for specific classes of drugs used for pain management.
- Discuss how use of adjuvant medications, such as antidepressants, anticonvulsants, anxiolytics, and sleep medications can be used most appropriately for pain management.
- Discuss how complementary techniques such as behavioral therapy, play therapy, and physical therapy can be utilized to manage pain and anxiety.
- Describe the role of the pediatric pain consultant/pain management team and discuss barriers to local availability.

SKILLS

Pediatric hospitalists should be able to:
- Accurately assess the presence and level of pain in children regardless of developmental level utilizing history, physical examination, physiologic parameters, and validated pediatric pain scales.
- Appropriately prescribe doses of analgesic medication that ameliorate pain while avoiding untoward side effects.
- Demonstrate proficiency in adjusting drug doses in the face of breakthrough pain.

- Safely prescribe equi-analgesic doses or adjust doses appropriately when changing from intravenous to oral therapy or when switching from one medication to another.
- Select and order pain and anxiety medications in safe and cost-effective manner.
- Correctly calculate and order a pain and anxiolytic medication tapering regimen that avoids withdrawal symptoms or breakthrough pain.
- Perform careful reassessments daily and as needed, note changes in clinical status, pain, side effects, and withdrawal symptoms and respond with appropriate actions.
- Order appropriate monitoring and correctly interpret monitor data.
- Anticipate and recognize potential side effects of analgesic and anxiolytic medications and respond with appropriate actions.
- Consistently utilize non-pharmacologic methods as part of a pain management plan.
- Identify patients likely to have chronic pain, and involve appropriate consultants to assist with long term management.
- Identify patients with neuropathic pain and develop a treatment plan with assistance from appropriate consultants.
- Correctly identify discharge needs and create a comprehensive discharge plan attending to equipment, medications, and specialty services required.

ATTITUDES

Pediatric hospitalists should be able to:
- Educate patients and the family/caregiver on various aspects of pain, including etiologies, management, and impact on the healing process.
- Involve the primary care provider in the therapeutic process early in the hospitalization and work together to coordinate appropriate follow-up care.
- Recognize the impact of uncontrolled pain has on patients' emotional and physical well-being.
- Collaborate with subspecialists and the primary care provider to ensure coordinated longitudinal care for children receiving chronic pain management services.

SYSTEMS ORGANIZATION AND IMPROVEMENT

In order to improve efficiency and quality within their organizations, pediatric hospitalists should:
- Work with hospital administration, hospital staff, subspecialists and others to implement a comprehensive, systematic approach to pain management across the continuum of care.
- Lead, coordinate or participate in the development and implementation of cost-effective, safe, evidence-based care to standardize the evaluation and management for hospitalized children with pain.
- Educate other healthcare providers who may work with children on pediatric pain assessment and safe medication use.
- Work in consultation with surgical staff to prioritize and improve the management of pain in pediatric surgical patients.

PEDIATRIC ADVANCED LIFE SUPPORT

INTRODUCTION

The American Academy of Pediatrics (AAP) and the American Heart Association (AHA), in conjunction with International Liaison Committee on Resuscitation (ILCOR), developed the Pediatric Advanced Life Support (PALS) curriculum. The course teaches healthcare providers to more effectively recognize potential respiratory failure and shock in infants and children and to respond with early appropriate interventions to prevent cardiopulmonary arrest. The hallmark of the PALS curriculum is the rapid identification of life threatening conditions in infants and children by utilizing a 4-tiered Pediatric Assessment scheme focused on simplicity and graduated to provoke timely and appropriate early interventions. The scheme uses a recurring cycle of "assess-categorize-decide-act" management scheme for the management of seriously ill or injured infants and children. This scheme funnels emergency decision making into respiratory (distress or failure) and circulatory (compensated or hypotensive) categories, which can be further defined, based upon additional information gathered in the 4-tiered assessment process. The PALS curriculum further emphasizes the importance of the Resuscitation Team Concept, which encourages clear, collaborative communication. The Neonatal Resuscitation Program (NRP), also offered by the AAP and AHA, addresses the resuscitation of the newborn in the delivery room or in the neonatal intensive care unit and is discussed elsewhere in this publication. Pediatric hospitalists frequently encounter clinical situations that require immediate intervention based on these guidelines.

KNOWLEDGE

Pediatric hospitalists should be able to:
- Define the roles, team composition, and responsibilities of "rapid response" and "code blue" teams, noting local context.
- List the common etiologies and recognize early signs of respiratory failure and all forms of shock, attending to variations in each due to age.
- Describe how deterioration can lead to cardiopulmonary arrest when early signs of distress are not recognized or acted upon.
- Discuss the utility of early warning systems/pediatric rapid assessment tools designed to anticipate significant clinical instability within the local context.
- Describe how basic airway, breathing, circulation, and disability, and exposure ("ABCDE") life support maneuvers differ with age from newborns to infants and older children.
- Summarize the modalities commonly available to support the airway, breathing and circulation in children with worsening respiratory distress, in increasing intensity/invasiveness.
- Compare and contrast the advantages, disadvantages, and proper selection of bag-mask ventilation versus advanced airway management techniques.
- Describe the pathophysiology of hypovolemic, septic, and cardiogenic shock.
- Review the approach toward stabilization of hypovolemic, septic and cardiogenic shock, attending to varied age groups and including treatments and testing.
- Explain how assessment tools and interventions should be customized for special resuscitation situations such as trauma, toxicological emergencies, rapid sequence intubation, procedural sedation, children with special health care needs and others.
- List common pediatric cardiac dysrhythmias and describe the most appropriate algorithm to apply for each.
- Describe the appropriate context and use of automated external defibrillators in children.
- Review the management of post resuscitation care and transport.
- Discuss the basic pharmacology of drugs most commonly utilized in PALS.

SKILLS

Pediatric hospitalists should be able to:
- Successfully complete the Pediatric Advanced Life Support course and maintain certification.
- Recognize early warning signs of acute respiratory distress and cardiac compromise and institute corrective actions to avert further deterioration.
- Identify patients requiring institution of PALS techniques, accurately perform rapid assessment, and apply appropriate interventions.
- Perform effective cardiopulmonary resuscitation and basic life support skills.
- Perform effective resuscitation and stabilization of newborns in the delivery room as appropriate for local context.
- Efficiently stabilize the airway, using effective non-invasive and invasive airway management techniques in collaboration with other services as appropriate.
- Efficiently obtain peripheral or central vascular access by placement if intravenous, intraosseous or central venous catheters in collaboration with other services as appropriate.
- Correctly identify and treat common pediatric cardiac dysrhythmias.
- Correctly utilize an Automated External Defibrillator under appropriate circumstances.
- Effectively use weight/size based resuscitation tools.
- Correctly apply PALS principles to special resuscitation situations such as toxicological emergencies, procedural sedation, or trauma.

ATTITUDES

Pediatric hospitalists should be able to:
- Effectively lead or participate as a member of a stabilization (rapid response) and/or resuscitation (code blue) team.
- Communicate effectively and compassionately with the family/caregiver.
- Advocate for family/caregiver presence during resuscitation when appropriate.
- Collaborate with the primary care provider to enhance support for the family/caregiver.

SYSTEMS ORGANIZATION AND IMPROVEMENT

In order to improve efficiency and quality within their organizations, pediatric hospitalists should:
- Lead, coordinate or participate in the development of a local Pediatric Advanced Life Support training program.
- Work with hospital administration to ensure code carts are pediatric-specific and contain adequate, appropriate equipment.
- Work with hospital administration to create inter-facility transport and affiliation agreements between community hospitals and pediatric tertiary care centers to foster effective and appropriate triage of sick and injured children.
- Advocate for statewide Emergency Medical Systems (EMS) for Children program which places pediatric emergency care in its proper place within the EMS system.

PROCEDURAL SEDATION

INTRODUCTION

Sedation is often used to minimize procedure related pain and to provide decreased motion for diagnostic studies. Control of pain, anxiety and memory may minimize negative psychological responses to treatment and also lead to a higher success rate for the therapy or diagnostic test. Safe attainment of these goals requires careful preparation and decision-making prior to the procedure, meticulous monitoring during the procedure, and application of skills to avoid or treat the complications of sedation including ability to rescue patients from a deeper level of sedation than intended. With appropriate training and experience, pediatric hospitalists can safely provide a range of sedation services for pediatric patients.

KNOWLEDGE

Pediatric hospitalists should be able to:
- Describe the goals of sedation, such as pain control, anxiolysis, amnesia, and motion control.
- List commonly used single or combinations of medications, and describe how each achieves the desired goal with the minimum risk of complications and side effects.
- Compare and contrast the goals of isolated anxiolysis with minimal sedation, attending to issues such as medication choice and dosing, procedure, and patient past procedural history.
- Define minimal sedation, moderate sedation, deep sedation, and general anesthesia as established by the American Society of Anesthesiologists (ASA), American Academy of Pediatrics (AAP), and The Joint Commission (TJC).
- Discuss the pharmacology and effects of commonly used sedation medications, including planned effects and potential side effects.
- Explain why non-pharmacologic interventions such as bundling, glucose water pacifiers, family/caregiver presence, visual imagery, deep breathing, music and others are important adjuncts to medication use in mitigating the perception of pain and anxiety.
- Explain the risks inherent with administration of sedating medications, and list the proper monitoring necessary to avoid or promptly recognize instability.
- Describe how age, disease process, and anatomy may increase the risk of sedation complications.
- Discuss the proper level of monitoring personnel necessary to maximize safety.
- Review indications for use of common reversal drugs, including anticipated results and duration of rescue effects.

SKILLS

Pediatric hospitalists should be able to:
- Perform a pre-sedation evaluation and appropriately assign ASA class and delineate patient-specific risks.
- Correctly recognize patients at higher risk and efficiently refer to an anesthesiologist.
- Correctly obtain informed consent from the family/caregiver.
- Develop a sedation plan that is based on the pre-sedation evaluation and considers goals for the sedation and risks to patients.
- Communicate effectively with the healthcare team before, during, and after the sedation to ensure that safe and efficient care is rendered.
- Identify complications and respond with appropriate actions.
- Manage the airway and provide pediatric advanced life support in case of known or unexpected complications.
- Order appropriate monitoring and correctly interpret monitor data.
- Identify when recovery criteria are met, and initiate an appropriate discharge/transfer plan.

ATTITUDES

Pediatric hospitalists should be able to:
- Work collaboratively with hospital staff and subspecialists to ensure coordinated planning and performance of sedation.
- Communicate effectively with patients and the family/caregiver regarding the indications for, risks, benefits, and steps of sedation.

SYSTEMS ORGANIZATION AND IMPROVEMENT

In order to improve efficiency and quality within their organizations, pediatric hospitalists should:
- Lead, coordinate or participate in the development and implementation of cost-effective, safe, evidence-based procedures and policies for performance of sedation for children.
- Lead, coordinate or participate in the development and implementation of a system for review of family/ caregiver and healthcare provider satisfaction into procedural strategies.
- Work with hospital staff and subspecialists to develop and implement management strategies for sedation.
- Lead, coordinate or participate in the development and implementation of a system for review of the efficacy, efficiency and outcomes of intravenous access procedures.
- Lead, coordinate or participate in the development and implementation of a system for review of the efficacy, efficiency and outcomes of sedation procedures.

RADIOGRAPHIC INTERPRETATION

INTRODUCTION

Radiographic studies are commonly performed throughout a wide range of pediatric healthcare settings. Imaging can play a pivotal role in the acute and chronic medical and surgical management of ill children. The explosion of imaging technology and expertise in the past three decades has resulted in an increased array of imaging modalities from which to choose. Access to and interpretation of imaging studies for children varies greatly between facilities. Pediatric hospitalists frequently encounter patients requiring imaging studies, and should be adept at ordering and interpreting images in collaboration with radiologist and other subspecialists.

KNOWLEDGE

Pediatric hospitalists should be able to:
- Review basic human anatomy and relate this to interpretation of common plain radiographs of areas such as the chest, abdomen, airway, and long bones.
- Describe the indications and limitations of the common radiographic modalities such as sonography, computed tomography, magnetic resonance imaging, plain radiography, and bone scans.
- Describe the risks of ionizing radiation in children and review the concept of ALARA (as low as reasonably achievable) in limiting radiation exposure.

- Review the indications for and benefits and risks of oral and intravenous contrast.
- Review the indications for anxiolysis, sedation, and anaesthesia attending to age, developmental stage, and procedure being performed.
- Compare and contrast indications for interventional radiologist versus general surgical consultation.
- Discuss the role of the radiologist as consultant.
- Discuss the appropriate imaging modality selection(s) for common emergent clinical presentations such as altered mental status, stridor, potential bowel obstruction, and others.
- Compare and contrast the utility, risks, and costs of different imaging modalities for presentations of complicated pneumonia and acute abdominal pain.

SKILLS

Pediatric hospitalists should be able to:
- Correctly determine the optimal study to answer a specific clinical question in a cost-effective manner, accounting for the limitations and risks of the study.
- Accurately order radiologic studies, noting indications for the study, sedation/anaesthesia need, and other relevant information in the order.
- Engage the radiologist as consultant as appropriate.
- Accurately interpret plain radiographs of the chest and abdomen for children 0-18 years of age.
- Correctly identify the need for and efficiently access interventional radiologists as appropriate.
- Communicate effectively with the healthcare team including radiologist and anaesthesiologist (as appropriate) to ensure safe, efficient and effective performance of radiologic studies.
- Correctly interpret and apply the results of radiographic studies into clinical care plans.

ATTITUDES

Pediatric hospitalists should be able to:
- Elicit and allay common family/caregiver concerns regarding radiation risks.
- Work collaboratively with hospital staff, radiologists, and anaesthesiologists to ensure coordinated planning and performance of radiologic studies.
- Communicate effectively with patients and the family/caregiver regarding the indications for, risks, benefits, and steps involved in the radiologic procedure.
- Recognize the importance of obtaining results of all studies and reviewing images in person whenever possible.

SYSTEMS ORGANIZATION AND IMPROVEMENT

In order to improve efficiency and quality within their organizations, pediatric hospitalists should:
- Lead, coordinate or participate in the development and implementation of cost-effective, safe, evidence-based standards for radiology services for children.
- Work with hospital administration to assure that a reliable and efficient radiographic imaging service is available for pediatric inpatients at the local facility.
- Lead, coordinate or participate in development and implementation of a system to review the accuracy of readings for pediatric patients and develop local criteria for tertiary referral center consultation.
- Collaborate with hospital administration and community partners to develop and sustain referral networks between local facilities and tertiary referral centers that enable review of appropriately selected pediatric images.
- Work with hospital administration, subspecialists, and others to review acquisition of new technologies and assess the impact on patient care.

Pediatric Hospital Medicine Core Competencies

Section Three: Specialized Clinical Services

CHILD ABUSE AND NEGLECT

INTRODUCTION

Child abuse or neglect is the physical, sexual or emotional maltreatment of children, by a caregiver or other adult, resulting in injury or illness. Approximately 1 million children per year are victims of abuse or neglect resulting in nearly 2000 fatalities per year. Pediatric hospitalists provide care for these victims by identifying, assessing, and treating injuries as well as ensuring the safety of these children and others in the household. Pediatric hospitalists fulfill varied roles depending on the local services available, but in all cases work collaboratively with social service agencies and legal authorities in situations of alleged abuse.

KNOWLEDGE

Pediatric hospitalists should be able to:

- Describe the aspects of the history or physical examination that should prompt an evaluation for child abuse or neglect including specific patterns consistent with abuse such as shaken baby syndrome, malnutrition, specific long bone fracture patterns, skin demarcations, and others.
- Identify circumstances that may be associated with an increased risk of child abuse such as poverty, family/caregiver stress and isolation, intimate partner violence, special needs children and substance abuse.
- Discuss the utility of radiological and laboratory studies in the evaluation of suspected child abuse.
- List and discuss different medical diseases which may mimic the presentation of child abuse and neglect.
- Discuss cultural differences in the treatment of ill children that may cause unusual physical examination findings such as coining.
- Discuss the relationship between developmental stages of children and how these are related to accidental injuries.
- Identify the requirements for and steps involved in mandatory reporting of suspected child abuse to the local or state child protective agencies.
- Describe state and local statutes defining child maltreatment.
- Explain the local processes involved in a hospital admission including methods and timing of consultations and screening exams for both physical abuse and sexual assault cases.
- Describe the role of various consultants who may be involved in an evaluation such as ophthalmology, radiology, hematology, genetics, neurology, surgery, neurosurgery, child abuse and protection team, trauma team, social services, child protective services, psychiatry and others.
- Discuss the importance of proper, objective written documentation in the medical record.
- Explain the role of pediatric hospitalists in providing testimony in court either as attending of record or as expert witness, as appropriate for the local context and training.
- List local community resources available for the family/caregiver and abused children such as foster care, receiving homes, support groups, safe houses, parenting courses, and others.

SKILLS

Pediatric hospitalists should be able to:

- Document and collect evidence in collaboration with abuse experts as appropriate for the local context.
- Recognize physical examination findings that are suggestive of child abuse or neglect.
- Evaluate children who are failing to thrive for psychosocial contributors to the malnutrition.
- Recognize abuse in children presenting with injury and unexplained symptoms such as Apparent Life Threatening Event.
- Recognize fracture types on radiographs that are suggestive of child abuse.
- Differentiate bruises, burns, and skin demarcations typically seen in abuse from those seen in unintentional injury such as accidental trauma, childhood rashes, or use of culturally acceptable therapies.
- Perform a fundoscopic examination to screen for retinal hemorrhages in children with suspected abusive head trauma.
- Access relevant consults effectively and efficiently.
- Report suspected abuse promptly and effectively.
- Obtain critical tests and imaging efficiently and safely.

- Coordinate care with subspecialists, the primary care provider and other services and arrange an appropriate multidisciplinary transition plan for hospital discharge including determination of the location and responsible party to whom the child will be discharged.

ATTITUDES

Pediatric hospitalists should be able to:
- Realize that child abuse occurs in all cultures, ethnicities and socioeconomic classes.
- Communicate in a sensitive, empathetic, unbiased, and ethical manner.
- Communicate effectively with patients, the family/caregiver, and healthcare providers regarding findings and care plans.
- Maintain professionalism when providing assessments of suspected abuse cases to law enforcement or social service agencies.
- Collaborate with subspecialists and the primary care provider to ensure coordinated longitudinal care for abused children.

SYSTEMS ORGANIZATION AND IMPROVEMENT

In order to improve efficiency and quality within their organizations, pediatric hospitalists should:
- Lead, coordinate or participate in the development and implementation of cost-effective, safe, evidence-based care pathways to standardize evaluation and management for hospitalized children with suspected abuse.
- Collaborate with hospital administration and community partners to develop and sustain referral networks between community based practices or hospitals, tertiary referral centers, social service agencies and legal agencies.

HOSPICE AND PALLIATIVE CARE

INTRODUCTION

Pediatric palliative and/or hospice care are increasingly important components of the continuum of care for hospitalized children. As both a philosophy and an organized method for delivering care, these approaches to care focus on the relief of physical, psychosocial, and spiritual suffering experienced by infants, children and adolescents and the family/caregiver who face a life-threatening condition. The guiding philosophy includes comfort and quality of life, while at the same time sustaining hope despite the likelihood of death. The goals of this type of care include enhancing choices, relieving pain and suffering and ensuring the best quality of care for the child and family/caregiver during the stages of living, dying and grief and bereavement. Care may be provided at home, in an inpatient hospice setting or within a traditional hospital setting. Palliative care services are most easily accessible in the traditional intensive care and hospital settings. Resources for treatment of dying children outside of these settings may be quite limited and vary by geographic location. Pediatric hospitalists therefore are often in the best position to provide both leadership and clinical roles for children requiring these services. Pediatric hospitalists should be able to access available palliative and hospice services and must be comfortable managing ethical dilemmas encountered in the inpatient setting related to care of the dying patient.

KNOWLEDGE

Pediatric hospitalists should be able to:
- Define the terms palliative and hospice care and describe the similarities and differences between them.
- Give examples of children who may be appropriate for hospice and palliative care services.
- Describe why pediatric hospice and palliative care are optimally provided by an interdisciplinary team consisting of a pediatrician, pediatric nurse, social worker, chaplain, home health aide, and others.
- Compare and contrast multidisciplinary with interdisciplinary team dynamics.
- Describe why the decision related to forgoing potentially life-sustaining treatments or the withdrawal of life support often are best made before a child becomes critically ill.
- Discuss the elements of a treatment plan for relief of suffering, including appropriate consultations (such as palliative care, pain service, physiatrists, and others) and therapies (such as complementary medicine, pain medications, and others).

- Explain how elements of palliative treatment and curative treatment may simultaneously occur during the course of treatment of a child's life limiting illness.
- Identify local, regional, and national resources for pediatric palliative and hospice care that are accessible to patients, the family/caregiver, and healthcare providers.
- Describe the role and composition of a hospital Ethics Committee as it relates to patient and family/caregiver decisions regarding end-of-life decisions.
- Describe the processes involved in writing "Allow Natural Death (AND)" orders, pronouncing a person dead, completing a death certificate, discussing autopsy and donor mandates and options, and accessing immediate support for family/caregiver and staff.

SKILLS

Pediatric hospitalists should be able to:
- Proactively identify opportunities for appropriate referral to and utilization of hospice and palliative care services.
- Communicate "bad news" effectively and provide opportunities for patients and the family/caregiver to be introduced to palliative care or hospice services when appropriate.
- Manage ethical dilemmas encountered in the inpatient setting related to care of the dying patient.
- Integrate cultural issues in discussions and management of end of life issues.
- Effectively adapt communication methods to varying age and developmental stages to assure understanding of chronic illness, death and dying.
- Recognize and manage pain and other common symptoms causing distress for patients and the family/caregiver at the end of life.
- Correctly prescribe medication and non-medication therapies in collaboration with appropriate consultants.

ATTITUDES

Pediatric hospitalists should be able to:
- Create awareness for the importance of pediatric palliative and hospice care.
- Demonstrate awareness and acceptance of palliative care approaches, which may include alternative and/or complementary medical therapies.
- Role model ethical behavior at all times.
- Identify personal attitudes toward end of life care from a physical, psychosocial and spiritual perspective.
- Recognize when personal perspective and bias may influence care for dying patients.
- Identify gaps in personal knowledge, skills and attitudes regarding palliative care and utilize opportunities for professional education to address them.
- Collaborate with the interdisciplinary team, subspecialists and the primary care provider to ensure coordinated longitudinal care for children receiving palliative or hospice services.

SYSTEMS ORGANIZATION AND IMPROVEMENT

In order to improve efficiency and quality within their organizations, pediatric hospitalists should:
- Engage in organizational efforts to provide pediatric hospice and palliative care education for interdisciplinary teams.
- Create or help sustain a pediatric perspective for hospital Ethics Committees.
- Collaborate with hospital administration and community partners to ensure efficient access to appropriate consultants necessary for success of these programs for children.
- Advocate for development of pediatric hospice and palliative care resources in their hospital and their community.

LEADING A HEALTHCARE TEAM

INTRODUCTION

Leading a pediatric inpatient healthcare team requires maintaining advanced current knowledge of diseases and healthcare systems. A leader must recognize, support and encourage active participation by all team members to attain the highest level of group performance while creating a positive work environment. A leader should set a strategic direction and motivate others to work towards defined goals. More patients are cared for in ambulatory settings. As a result, pediatric patients who are admitted to the hospital often have more complex diseases or are more acutely ill. Children with special healthcare needs comprise more of the inpatient pediatric population. Care must be coordinated in an efficient, effective, and safe manner both during the hospital phase of care and at transitions of care. Pediatric hospitalists need to develop leadership skills to assure care is rendered in a collaborative and interdisciplinary manner.

KNOWLEDGE

Pediatric hospitalists should be able to:
- Distinguish between the goals, methods, and styles of a leader and those of a manager.
- Describe methods used to strengthen leadership skills, such as role playing or attendance at leadership conferences.
- State the importance of clear communication between all members of the healthcare team when collaborating to care for children.
- Give examples of skills needed to be an effective team leader, including critical thinking, evidence-based decision-making, and use of continuous quality improvement principles.
- Compare and contrast potential healthcare team members in various settings such as community, tertiary care, academic, and non-academic.
- Discuss pediatric hospitalists' role as team leader in coordination of care, particularly where other physician subspecialists are involved in co-management.
- List issues that impact team dynamics, such as personalities, perceptions, and varied individual clinical skills of team members.
- Recognize how conflict or enmeshment can be created within a team or between team members and patients and the family/caregiver.
- Articulate the skills needed to lead a healthcare team that includes trainees.
- Describe methods that enhance team efficiency.
- Explain the roles of key personnel, facilities, and equipment in various clinical settings.
- Define the team relationship between pediatric hospitalists, the primary care provider, patients and the family/caregiver in the context of the medical home and family centered care.
- Define terms related to documentation, billing and coding such as compliance, Relative Value Units (RVUs) and authorizations and articulate why it is important for healthcare team members to understand them.

SKILLS

Pediatric hospitalists should be able to:
- Lead family-centered rounds in an effective manner promoting communication and participation by team members.
- Maintain strong diagnostic and relevant procedure skills and be able to provide mentorship in these skills.
- Lead patient throughput in a way that optimizes bed flow and care.
- Maintain proficiency in administrative skills such as documentation, billing and coding compliance, RVU collection, and contracting and mentor other team members in attaining these skills.
- Demonstrate excellent communication skills, including expressive and listening ability, in all interactions with other members of the healthcare team.
- Build consensus within the health care team on evidence-based care management algorithms, hospital policies and related issues.
- Identify when healthcare team members may have a conflict affecting patient care delivery and offer appropriate support in a discrete manner.
- Delegate team responsibilities in an effective and equitable manner.
- Deal constructively in managing conflicts with and among supervisors, staff, and trainees, seeking resolutions that promote productivity and good will.
- Effect systems change through use of quality improvement tools such as Plan-Do-Study-Act (PDSA), Failure Mode Effects Analysis (FMEA) and others.
- Establish skills in time management.
- Run an effective meeting to accomplish outlined goals in a defined time period.

ATTITUDES

Pediatric hospitalists should be able to:
- Demonstrate a consistent level of commitment, responsibility, and accountability in rendering patient care.
- Consistently display honesty, integrity, humility, and fairness in working with patients and the family/caregiver, and all members of the healthcare team.
- Respect the skills and contributions of all members of the healthcare team.
- Pursue continued development of leadership skills through additional training opportunities.
- Maintain a professional manner at all times.

SYSTEMS ORGANIZATION AND IMPROVEMENT

In order to improve efficiency and quality in their organizations, pediatric hospitalists should:
- Identify and work to resolve barriers to teamwork between healthcare professionals.
- Lead interdisciplinary collaboration at the bedside to promote patient safety, quality improvement, and cost-effective care for children.
- Proactively work to assure the healthcare team integrates and sustains family centered care principles.

NEWBORN CARE AND DELIVERY ROOM MANAGEMENT
INTRODUCTION

Pediatric hospitalists are often asked to support delivery and newborn services. For those who provide these services, the components vary and may include any combination of normal newborn examination and discharge, emergency delivery care, level II neonatal intensive care stabilization, level II neonatal care, or neonatal intensive care transport services. Rendering this care requires medical and procedural skills, as well as leadership and team skills while working with obstetricians, nurses, nurse midwives, advanced practice nurses, primary care providers, neonatologists, and families. Pediatric hospitalists are well positioned to provide care for the immediate newborn and assure effective transition of care at transport or discharge home.

KNOWLEDGE

Pediatric hospitalists should be able to:
- Describe the role of each team member commonly involved in newborn care, including the obstetrician, prenatal ultrasonographers/radiologists, primary care providers, nurses, lactation consultants, and others.
- Review the basic physiologic differences between the preterm and term infant, attending to cardiopulmonary needs, respiratory control, feeding issues, and other elements.
- Discuss the impact of maternal factors on the fetus and newborn, including abnormal pre-natal labs, maternal diabetes, thyroid disorders, and prescription, non-prescription and illicit drug use.
- Define nursery care levels and give an example of infants should be cared for at each level.
- Describe the normal delivery process and the physiologic transitions of a newborn infant.
- Describe the skills needed to be an effective resuscitation team leader, including critical thinking, evidence-based decision-making, and use of continuous quality improvement principles.
- Describe the benefits of breast milk, formulas and supplements (Vitamin D, Iron) in infant nutrition for term and preterm infants.
- Review the components of newborn screening, and state which tests are performed locally.
- Discuss factors influencing bilirubin levels and summarize current guidelines for treatment of jaundice.
- Review guidelines for common neonatal care such as immunizations, Vitamin K, eye prophylaxis, hearing screening, car seat trials and electrolyte and bilirubin screening.
- Discuss the role of maternal group B streptococcal screen, and presence or absence of chorioamnionitis in the management of the newborn.
- Describe the diagnostic and therapeutic approach toward newborns with common dysmorphisms, including features associated with trisomies, ear pits, cleft-lip/palate, supranummary digits, and clubfoot.

- Describe the approach toward the diagnosis and treatment of common infections and toxic exposures of newborns.
- Describe the pathophysiology of persistent fetal circulation/pulmonary hypertension.
- Describe stabilization techniques and list the differential diagnoses for newborns with seizures.
- Review the role of pre-natal ultrasounds and describe appropriate post-birth follow-up of common findings, such as umbilical cord anomalies, renal abnormalities and heart lesions.
- List the clinical indications for an acute metabolic or endocrine work-up in newborns.
- Compare and contrast the characteristics of benign versus pathologic cardiac murmurs, and describe the role of oxygen saturation testing.
- Discuss the appropriate interventions for a cardiac murmur, including indications for and timing of cardiology consultation
- Describe the elements of a safe discharge, attending to timing and follow-up plans.

SKILLS

Pediatric hospitalists should be able to:
- Maintain Neonatal Resuscitation Program (NRP) certification.
- Provide care that incorporates current best practices for oxygen at delivery, infant warming, and treatment of asphyxia.
- Correctly order and manage enteral and parenteral nutrition for neonates.
- Perform a comprehensive exam and document normal and abnormal variants, including complications of delivery.
- Initiate an NRP-based infant resuscitation, effectively leading the team in the resuscitation of an extremely premature to term infant.
- Provide leadership for a normal newborn or level II nursery in partnership with neonatologists and other subspecialists as indicated.
- Identify infants with respiratory and cardiac problems and appropriately initiate cardiorespiratory support.
- Accurately perform procedures such as lumbar puncture, placement of enteral tubes, umbilical catheters, venous access, intraosseous placement, exchange transfusion and needle thoracotomy or chest tube placement.
- Correctly identify newborns requiring subspecialty consultation and counseling such as those with ambiguous genitalia, dysmorphisms, and others and effectively coordinate the referral and subsequent care as indicated.
- Recognize and provide initial care for newborns with surgical emergencies, such as infants with gastrointestinal obstruction, diaphragmatic hernia, and others.

ATTITUDES

Pediatric hospitalists should be able to:
- Demonstrate a consistent level of commitment, responsibility, and accountability in rendering patient care for newborns
- Role model professional behavior, demonstrating compassion for women and families during the delivery process, when discussing care options, and consultation or referral need, as indicated.
- Communicate effectively with patients, the family/caregiver and healthcare providers regarding findings and care plans including post-discharge needs.
- Recognize and respect decisions of the family/caregiver regarding care of extremely premature infants or infants with anomalies.

SYSTEMS ORGANIZATION AND IMPROVEMENT

In order to improve efficiency and quality in their organizations, pediatric hospitalists should:
- Lead, coordinate or participate in the development and implementation of cost-effective, evidence-based care pathways to standardize the evaluation, management and discharge process for newborns.
- Work with hospital administration, hospital staff, subspecialists, and other services/consultants to provide appropriate newborn resuscitation services.
- Collaborate with hospital administration and community partners to develop and sustain referral networks between local facilities and tertiary referral centers for newborns requiring tertiary care.

TECHNOLOGY DEPENDENT CHILDREN

INTRODUCTION

The last several decades have seen a surge in the number of children with special health care needs, currently estimated to account for 13% of all children and for 70% of all child health care expenditures. Many of these children require some form of technological assistance to compensate for loss or impairment of one or more vital functions. Advances in intensive care practices and improved survival have resulted in an increase in the number and complexity of technology dependent infants and children being cared for both on acute inpatient floors and at home. Commonly used devices include gastrostomy and jejunostomy tubes with and without fundoplication, ventricular shunts, baclofen pumps, indwelling central venous catheters, tracheostomies, and various forms of non-invasive ventilation. Pediatric hospitalists frequently encounter these technology dependent children, and therefore must have a working knowledge of the these devices and technologies, as well as an understanding of the associated challenges that may arise both in and out of the hospital and within the continuum of the child's life. Care coordination for these children has been reported to result in clinical and process improvements, reduced health care costs, and improved family/caregiver satisfaction. The importance of these issues is reflected in the work of the National Center of Medical Home Initiatives for Children with Special Needs and in an American Academy of Pediatrics policy statement, "The Medical Home."

KNOWLEDGE

Pediatric hospitalists should be able to:

- List the indications for placement and removal of common enteral feeding devices such as nasogastric, nasojejunal, percutaneous gastrostomy, surgically performed gastrostomy tube with and without fundoplication, and gastro-jejunal tube.
- Discuss the utility of evaluation techniques for disorders that may require these interventions, attending to therapist, developmental, and radiographic evaluations.
- Compare and contrast the risks, benefits, and alternatives of various modes of long term intravenous access and externally implanted, totally implanted, and percutaneously implanted catheter types such as Broviac, Mediport, PICC and others.
- Discuss the medical and ethical considerations for the initiation and removal of chronic respiratory support, including interventions such as tracheostomy, bilevel positive airway pressure, continuous positive airway pressure, and others.
- Review common acute problems relating to specific medical devices, such as central venous catheter infection and enteral feeding tube dysfunction, and discuss the diagnostic evaluation and treatment of these problems.
- Compare and contrast nosocomial infection risk in patients chronically dependent on technology compared to hospitalized patients with acute, limited technology device use.
- State how the National Patient Safety Goals relate to the care of these patients, and describe how best practices around these goals are applied when rendering care.
- Summarize how common acute systemic illnesses affect the technology dependent child from both short and long term perspectives.
- Define pain, anxiety, fear, and depression in patients undergoing evaluation or manipulation of medical devices and explain the interrelationship between them.
- Describe the social, emotional and fiscal impact of assessment, initiation, and/or removal of medical devices on the family/caregiver.
- Discuss the technical and practical aspects of homecare delivery for technology dependent children and the family/caregiver.
- Describe issues or concerns which should prompt referrals to the ethics committee, hospice, or palliative care services.
- List the community and educational resources for technology dependent children.

SKILLS

Pediatric hospitalists should be able to:

- Create a comprehensive discharge plan including device care and explicit emergency response instructions for the family/caregiver.
- Coordinate care with subspecialists and the primary care provider maintaining the medical home model.

- Write a comprehensive yet succinct summary appeal letter to insurers if medically indicated services are denied.
- Demonstrate clinical proficiency in basic care of common medical devices as well as emergency management of common complications such as accidental tracheostomy decannulation or gastrostomy tube extrusion.
- Clinically evaluate fit and function of devices, attending to the child's age and developmental stage.
- Implement and adjust common medications used in conjunction with medical devices.
- Coordinate end-of-life interdisciplinary discussions between appropriate subspecialists, teams, primary care provider, and the family/caregiver, and implement this care when appropriate.

ATTITUDES

Pediatric hospitalists should be able to:
- Provide leadership to an interdisciplinary team, reflecting awareness that hospitalization is a phase of longitudinal care.
- Model communication skills that are clear, compassionate, and sensitive to religious and cultural values of patients and the family/caregiver.
- Advocate for medically-appropriate devices and the support services necessary to maintain these.
- Recognize the need to continually assess patient and family/caregiver needs relating to technology dependence within the context of developmental and quality of life concerns.
- Collaborate with subspecialists and the primary care provider to ensure coordinated longitudinal care for technology dependent children.

SYSTEMS ORGANIZATION AND IMPROVEMENT

In order to improve efficiency and quality within their organizations, pediatric hospitalists should:
- Lead, coordinate or participate in the development and implementation of systems within the hospital to ensure comprehensive patient and family/caregiver-centered care for the technology dependent child.
- Lead, coordinate or participate in quality improvement initiatives to improve care for the technology dependent child.
- Collaborate with local, state, and national political groups to educate and champion for equitable access to current technology for all of these children, and for research funding to enhance their future.

TRANSPORT OF THE CRITICALLY ILL CHILD

INTRODUCTION

Pediatric inter-facility transport first began in the 1970s when a two-fold difference in mortality was first demonstrated between neonates cared for solely at a community hospital versus those transferred to a regional center. Today as medicine continues to make technological strides and therapeutic advances, community hospitals often find themselves ill equipped to provide acute care to ill and injured children. The growing trend toward centralized pediatric services further necessitates the transfer of children requiring subspecialty care to a regional facility. From these forces has come the advent of the pediatric critical care transport service. Like their neonatal counterparts, pediatric critical care transport teams are overseen in large part by pediatric intensivists or emergency medicine physicians. However, increasing demand for transport of non-critically ill children, increasing presence of pediatric hospitalists, and increasing time constraints felt by pediatric intensivists is shifting the paradigm. Co-direction of pediatric critical care transport services by intensivists and hospitalists is becoming more common. Transport systems vary from institution to institution, some having a dedicated in-house pediatric critical care transport teams and others utilizing outside transport services. For transported patients, pediatric hospitalists may serve as referring or accepting attending physician, transport physician, or transport coordinator. Through each of these roles pediatric hospitalists fulfill an essential function in ensuring the safe and timely transport of ill children.

KNOWLEDGE

Pediatric hospitalists should be able to:
- Compare and contrast advantages and disadvantages between transport modalities including non-medical, Basic Life Support (BLS) ambulance, Advanced Life Support (ALS) ambulance, Critical Care Team (CCT) ambulance, and specialized Neonatal/Pediatric Critical Care Transport service (Table 1).

- Discuss the role of the transport coordinator in effectively triaging to the proper facility, engaging subspecialty services, and determining safest modality of transport.
- List the critical history and physical examination elements necessary (to give or obtain) to ensure a safe, effective, expeditious transport, attending to verbal, written, and electronic formats.
- Explain how the selection of mode of transportation and team composition are influenced by patients' clinical status and transport logistics such as local traffic conditions, geographical distance, weather, and resources (internal and external) available at the time of the transport.
- Describe the role of subspecialist and intensivist consultation in stabilization and management during transport and upon arrival to the destination facility.
- Describe the knowledge base and skill set of non-physician transport team members.
- Review the use of standardized procedures on transport, including how they are used by non-physician team members and the process for creation, approval, and oversight.
- Discuss basic altitude physiology and describe how clinical conditions such as hypoxia can be impacted by changes in altitude.
- Summarize the transport process, including communications, documentation, and team member roles attending to local context.
- Discuss the role of the transport program in the local community, including services provided and outreach education.

SKILLS

Pediatric hospitalists should be able to*:
(*As appropriate for pediatric hospitalists' role as referring or accepting attending physician, transport physician, or transport coordinator.)

- Efficiently obtain or give critical clinical information placing particular emphasis on cardiac, pulmonary, and neurologic disease that could impact the transport process.
- Provide recommendations regarding laboratory studies and imaging, as well as therapeutic options for referring facilities and physicians.
- Effectively prepare the team to anticipate possible complications during any point in the transport, communicating all available clinical information and creating action plans for potential complications prior to transport.
- Manage care during transport at a level and quality of care equivalent to that offered in the acute care hospital setting, limited only by medications and services not available during transport.
- Demonstrate strong clinical abilities and expertise over a wide range of pediatric disease processes, making rapid assessments and initiating action plans on transport or at the referring or receiving facility.
- Stabilize or remotely direct stabilization of patients at the referring facility and on transport, appropriately utilizing current Pediatric Advanced Life Support guidelines.
- Obtain training and maintain skills for transport coordination, referral, and acceptance, including specialized transport issues such as flight physiology as appropriate.
- Where pediatric hospitalists' roles include participation in neonatal transport, appropriately utilize current Neonatal Resuscitation Program and STABLE Program guidelines.
- Recognize when to consult subspecialist, intensivist, or surgeon.
- Accurately document actions and discussions in the medical record.

ATTITUDES

Pediatric hospitalists should be able to:
- Respond promptly and courteously to all calls and requests for transport.
- Participate in educational programs for transport team members and community referral sources.
- Provide mentorship to junior hospitalists on all aspects of transport including clinical decision making, risk management, customer service, and operational issues.
- Communicate effectively with patients and the family/caregiver regarding the need for and their role in the transport, as appropriate.
- Establish and maintain good working relationships with referral sources and transport team members.

- Recognize and manage patient care related conflicts among transport team members or referring facility in a prompt and judicious manner.

SYSTEMS ORGANIZATION AND IMPROVEMENT

In order to improve efficiency and quality within their organizations, pediatric hospitalists should:
- Work with hospital administration, transport team members, and specifically with the transport program manager, on the growth and development of the pediatric transport service and or policies.
- Lead, coordinate or participate in ongoing educational opportunities to maintain the skill set of team members and transport coordinators.
- Lead, coordinate or participate in the development and implementation of cost-effective, safe, evidence-based care pathways to standardize the management of common diagnoses for children transported between facilities.
- Lead, coordinate or participate in establishing a multidisciplinary forum such as morbidity and mortality conference to regularly review cases with a goal of improving system-wide processes and outcomes.

TABLE 1. Options for Pediatric Inter-facility Transport (may vary according to local and regional resources)

Transport Modality	Advantage	Disadvantage
Non-medical (family/ caregiver)	Low cost.	No ability to intervene as condition deteriorates. Transport may be delayed due to detours or misdirection.
BLS Ambulance or volunteer ambulance	Emergency Medical Technician escort. Some ability to intervene if condition deteriorates.	Little to no pediatric experience thus interventions are limited. Transport may be delayed due to variable ambulance availability.
ALS Ambulance or mid-level transport	Paramedic escort; 1500-2000 hours of medical training, including O2 administration, nebulized medications, ALS, and airway skills. Greater ability to triage and intervene if condition deteriorates.	Pediatric training not uniform. Paramedics primarily trained for extrication, intervention and rapid transport.
CCT ambulance	Critical care nurse team member. Allows for higher level of assessment and intervention.	Pediatric expertise is uncommon.
Specialized pediatric-neonatal critical care transport service	2-3 member team composed of RN and RT (pediatric/neonatal critical care) and physician (hospital or emergency medicine, intensivist). Specialized pediatric assessment, monitoring, diagnostic, and interventional skills allows for high level pediatric care from initial referral.	High cost, limited resources.

Pediatric Hospital Medicine Core Competencies

Section Four: Healthcare Systems:
Supporting and Advancing Child Health

ADVOCACY

INTRODUCTION

Advocacy is defined as the process of speaking out in support of a specific individual, cause or program as distinct from the direct provision of material support to the individual, cause or program. In pediatric hospital medicine, advocacy can occur as an isolated event for a single patient, but is most effective when it leads to a change in an approach to a problem that supports multiple individuals in similar circumstances. Advocacy skills are part of the toolkit of both physicians and leaders. In conjunction with other healthcare professionals and organizations, pediatric hospitalists have an important role to play in advocating for both the children and the evolving field of hospital medicine. Pediatric hospitalists may also be called upon to advocate for the pediatric services or department within the hospital, as well as for children in the community.

KNOWLEDGE

Pediatric hospitalists should be able to:
- Define advocacy and health policy.
- Describe how advocacy impacts the care of children both in the hospital and the community.
- Discuss the multiple levels of advocacy, including individual, group, institutional, community, and legislative advocacy.
- Illustrate how financing of child health relates to advocacy.
- Describe the relationship between pediatric quality and advocacy.
- Discuss the various areas of focus for advocacy efforts, including disease process/diagnosis, age group, socio-economic, cultural or demographic group, health systems, payment systems, and government or community agencies.
- Describe the legislative process and identify specific ways in which physicians can participate in this process to improve the health of children, especially those requiring hospitalization.
- List the key national organizations (such as the American Academy of Pediatrics, the Society of Hospital Medicine and National Association of Children's Hospitals and Related Institutions and others) with which pediatric hospitalists work to advocate for hospitalized pediatric patients
- Explain how private and governmental funding and oversight organizations (such as Leapfrog, Medicaid, The Joint Commission and many others) influence advocacy efforts for children's healthcare.
- Identify community characteristics, demographics, needs, and assets that impact children's healthcare, including the availability of social, educational, and medical services for children and the family/caregiver.
- State common barriers, especially those unique to the pediatric population, that impact hospital care for children.
- Cite advocacy efforts that are unique to community hospitals such as obtaining pediatric representation on key committees, establishing a relationship with a pediatric referral center, and developing relationships with adult subspecialists.
- Cite unique opportunities for advocacy in children's hospitals.
- Define the medical home and understand the role of pediatric hospitalists in delivering care within a medical home.

SKILLS

Pediatric hospitalists should be able to:
- Conduct effective family centered, interdisciplinary rounds.
- Consistently engage patients and the family/caregiver in medical-decision making.
- Deliver family-centered, comprehensive, coordinated care for medically complex children and other special populations.
- Develop collaborative relationships with other pediatric healthcare providers to advocate for children within the medical home model.
- Provide effective media interviews on relevant topics in various formats (such as print, radio, television, and other).
- Define, articulate, and gain support for the unique health care needs of children in the hospital setting as well as the community.

- Identify hospital environments or processes that lack a focus on children and take appropriate steps to advocate for pediatric-specific needs.
- Participate in the advocacy and health policy activities sponsored by local, community, and national organizations.

ATTITUDES

Pediatric hospitalists should be able to:
- Accept responsibility for child health advocacy.
- Recognize the cultural beliefs and biases of patients, family/caregiver, and healthcare providers and adapt to advocate for patients' needs.
- Realize that the most effective advocacy involves creation of coalitions and teams.
- Maintain awareness of political, cultural, and socio-economic factors affecting children's healthcare and the practice of pediatric hospital medicine.

SYSTEMS ORGANIZATION AND IMPROVEMENT

In order to improve efficiency and quality within their organizations and their communities, pediatric hospitalists should:
- Incorporate the institution's mission and vision statements into daily work.
- Work with key hospital leaders to assure child advocacy is fully integrated into the delivery of care on a daily basis.
- Establish effective relationships with hospital leaders, community leaders and local politicians to target a specific issue and/or serve as an expert pediatric consultant.
- Participate in the development of systems of care in your institution and beyond that promote effective care for hospitalized children.

BUSINESS PRACTICES

INTRODUCTION

Sound business practices form a foundation for the growth and effective development of pediatric hospital medicine programs. Business practice refers to program development and growth, practice management, contract negotiation, and financial solvency. Pediatric hospitalists require fundamental business skills to enhance individual success, and facilitate growth and stability of groups, divisions, and institutions. Hospitals increasingly need physician leaders with these skills to improve operational efficiency and meet other institutional needs. Pediatric hospitalists must acquire and maintain business skills that support the ability to negotiate and define hospitalist roles within the hospital, expand practices intelligently, anticipate and respond to change, and sustain financial success.

KNOWLEDGE

Pediatric hospitalists should be able to:
- Explain why clinical practice is a business that needs a sound business plan, professional management, and strategic planning. Discuss the elements of mission and vision statements.
- Identify institutional financial power structures and how resources are developed to build and sustain academic and non-academic programs.
- Compare and contrast the basic structure of hospital-employed and private practice pediatric hospital medicine models.
- Define the basic components assessed during the initial planning for a pediatric hospitalist practice, such as baseline and projected census, projected revenue and expenses, and impact on current and future stakeholders.
- Articulate the requirements for compliant billing and documenting when collaborating with physician extenders.
- Discuss the impact of critical practice variables on creation of an effective and efficient staffing plan, including:
  - Anticipated census, patient acuity and length of stay
  - Anticipated revenue streams and volume

  o Need for night and/or weekend coverage
  o Physician-to-patient ratios
- Compare and contrast pediatric hospitalist staffing models, including:
  o Rounding or patient-based model
  o Shift-based model
- List potential sources of non-clinical responsibilities, such as teaching, committee participation, administrative work, and research. Describe the impact of each on staffing models and revenue.
- Distinguish between various pediatric hospitalist compensation structures, including full salary, incentive salary, and case rate models.
- Define the Relative Value Unit (RVU) and its utility in tracking revenue and physician compensation.
- Discuss the difference between costs versus charges.
- Compare and contrast basic billing methods and revenue sources for the provider versus the hospital, and review the effect of payor mix on these.
- Articulate the importance of billing and coding compliance as it relates to physician compensation and physician-hospital contracting.
- Identify key elements of compliance monitored by the Office of the Inspector General (OIG) of the Department of Health and Human Services (DHHS).
- State the importance of professional credentialing, licensing and liability coverage.
- Describe key features of care management organizations, such as capitation, carve-outs, withholds, case-, disease-, and demand-management and their role in promoting quality of care and cost-control.

SKILLS

Pediatric hospitalists should be able to:
- Review basic business data including revenue, expenses, staff and marketing costs, and accounts receivable.
- Demonstrate basic negotiation skills through role play or attendance at negotiation sessions with third party payors, the institution, department chair, or other contracted entity.
- Consistently document in the medical record in a manner that meets expectations for billing and coding and for external certifying agencies.
- Effectively utilize a clinical documentation system with an emphasis on:
  o Efficient, accurate, and complete documentation to support coding and billing
  o Compliance with the Health Insurance Portability and Accountability Act of 1996 (HIPAA)
  o Compliance with trainee documentation guidelines, where applicable
- Complete coding and billing processes efficiently and accurately.
- Participate in group, division, and/or institutional business and finance committees.

ATTITUDES

Pediatric hospitalists should be able to:
- Advocate for a business model that encourages retention of pediatric hospitalists and allows for adequate staffing to support patient safety, and physician wellness.
- Role model accountability with regard to billing, coding and business regulations.
- Support the business of pediatric hospitalists, by maintaining fiscally awareness and proactively managing stakeholder expectations.
- Seek opportunities to acquire basic business skills.

SYSTEMS ORGANIZATION AND IMPROVEMENT

In order to improve efficiency and quality in their organizations, pediatric hospitalists should:
- Collaborate with colleagues and business office leaders to make sound group/division business decisions using performance feedback, peer review and quality improvement information.
- Engage with hospital administrators on strategic business planning, wherever possible.

COMMUNICATION

INTRODUCTION

Communication is defined as any process in which a message containing information is transferred, especially from one person to another, via any of a number of media. Communication may be delivered verbally or non-verbally, directly, (as in face-to-face conversation or with the observation of a gesture) or remotely, spanning space and time (as in writing, reading, making or playing back a recording, or using a computer). Pediatric hospitalists must be effective communicators in many venues such as when rendering direct patient care, performing hospital committee work, or educating trainees. However, the most important of these is the verbal communication that occurs at the bedside with patients, family/caregiver, and healthcare team. Successful patient care is elusive or wanting without proper communication.

KNOWLEDGE

Pediatric hospitalists should be able to:
- Compare and contrast the importance of listening and speaking for effective communication.
- Define the components of effective expressive and receptive (listening) communication, such as introduction of team members, avoiding medical jargon, tone, word choice, allowing time for patients and the family/caregiver to speak, and body language.
- List examples of common non-listening behaviors such as allowing distractions, asking unrelated questions, jumping to conclusions, interrupting the speaker, and failing to notice the speaker's non-verbal language.
- Cite methods that can be used when faced with difficult behaviors during communication, such as asking for a behavior change and paraphrasing to diffuse emotion.
- Describe patients in a cultural and spiritual context.
- Explain how vulnerabilities, life situation, limitation in activities of daily living, education, language and other factors should each be addressed when communicating with patients and the family/caregiver.
- Identify personal values, biases, skills, and relationships that may influence communication.
- Discuss the significance of including the family/caregiver and others who are most important to patients in patient care discussions.
- Explain why effective communication is central to patient care handoffs and list examples of best methods for communication both within hospitalist groups and with other healthcare providers.
- Articulate how to give bad news by expressing empathy, giving patients and the family/caregiver time to ask questions, maintaining calm, and choosing a quiet, private location for the discussion.
- Cite important features of effective written communication.
- Compare and contrast specific examples of effective and ineffective written communication, including timing of entries, legibility, disagreements on patient care decisions, documentation of changes in clinical status and others.

SKILLS

Pediatric hospitalists should be able to:
- Demonstrate command of a comprehensive array of expressive and receptive communication skills.
- Coordinate discussions with all caregivers to ensure a single clear message is given to patients and the family/caregiver.
- Actively participate in conflict resolution.
- Summarize the entire process and sequence of care for patients and the family/caregiver in understandable terms following the principles of family centered care.
- Maintain concise, complete written records that meet expectations of external reviewing agencies and malpractice carriers.
- Develop and implement a plan for daily communication that is family centered.

ATTITUDES

Pediatric hospitalists should be able to:
- Respect the skills and contributions of all involved in the care of patients.
- Exemplify professionalism in all communications.
- Seek opportunities to enhance communication skills.

SYSTEMS ORGANIZATION AND IMPROVEMENT

In order to improve efficiency and quality within their organizations, pediatric hospitalists should:
- Collaborate with hospital administrators to improve medical record documentation systems by technical means.
- Assist in the development of and/or participate in hospital and system-wide educational programs on communication skills.

CONTINUOUS QUALITY IMPROVEMENT

INTRODUCTION

Continuous Quality Improvement (CQI) in Health Care is a structured organizational process that involves physicians and other personnel in planning and implementing ongoing proactive improvements in processes of care to provide quality health care outcomes. CQI is used by hospitals to optimize clinical care by reducing variability and reducing costs, to help meet regulatory requirements, and to enhance customer service quality. The issues of quality improvement gained additional national attention with the 2001 release of the Institute of Medicine (IOM) report titled "Crossing the Quality Chasm" in which the template was set for quality improvement processes. Pediatric hospitalists are well positioned to promote and champion CQI projects within the hospital setting, working on the "front lines" of clinical care and acting as influential change agents.

KNOWLEDGE

Pediatric hospitalists should be able to:
- Distinguish the basic principles of CQI, which focus upon proactively improving processes of care, from Quality Assurance which focuses on conformance quality.
- Explain how CQI focuses on systematic improvement and can be effectively used to create clinical care plans as well as hospital procedural guidelines.
- Describe the business case for quality, and how quality drives cost.
- Discuss the CQI concept of and methods behind Plan Do Study Act (PDSA) and other models to accomplish rapid cycle improvements within the organization.
- List common terms and language of CQI and Performance Improvement.
- Define commonly used quality terms such as common cause and special cause variation, run charts, cumulative proportion charts, process measures, outcomes, and others.
- Explain the role of reliability science and human factors in implementing healthcare improvements.
- Summarize how CQI supports effective development of care standardization, best practices, and practice guidelines.
- Indicate how evidence-based medicine can be integrated into the CQI planning stage for appropriate clinical projects.
- Explain why building CQI into everyday processes of care is the most effective way to improve quality.
- Describe how decreasing unwanted variability in care impacts clinical outcomes.
- List the attributes necessary to moderate, facilitate and lead QI and patient safety initiatives and discuss the importance of team building methods.
- Describe the components of family centered care and discuss the importance of engaging patients and the family/caregiver in QI efforts.
- Identify the principles outlined in the IOM "Crossing the Quality Chasm" report and stay current with the latest IOM reports on hospital quality.
- Describe how external agencies and societies such as The Joint Commission , Child Health Corporation of America, National Association for Children's Hospitals and Related Institutions, Agency for Healthcare Research and Quality, and the National Quality Forum impact quality improvement initiatives for hospitalized children.
- Discuss the value of national, state, and local comparative quality data and the utility of national sources such as the Pediatric Health Information Dataset (PHIS).
- Describe the quality improvement education expectations of residency programs set by the ACGME and compare and contrast these to those of the American Board of Pediatrics.

SKILLS

Pediatric hospitalists should be able to:
- Lead as a physician champion and "early adopter" of continuous quality improvement.
- Participate in reviews of quality data, including basic data analysis and development of recommendations from the data.
- Serve as a liaison between physician staff and hospital administrative staff when interpreting physician-specific information and clinical care outliers.
- Initiate a continuous quality improvement project by identifying a process in need of improvement and engaging the appropriate personnel to implement a change, using CQI principles.
- Educate trainees, nursing staff, ancillary staff, peers on the basic principles of CQI and the importance of CQI on child health outcomes.
- Assist with development of best practices and practice guidelines to assure consistent, high quality standards and expectations for care in the hospital setting.
- Effectively use best practice guidelines.
- Demonstrate proficiency in performing a rapid cycle improvement project utilizing the PDSA process.
- Demonstrate facility with the use of common computer applications, including spreadsheet and database management for information retrieval and analysis.
- Effectively collaborate with appropriate healthcare providers critical to quality improvement efforts such as clinical team members, information technology staff, data analysts, and others.

ATTITUDES

Pediatric hospitalists should be able to:
- Lead as an "early adopter" and "change agent" by building an awareness of and consensus for changes needed to make patient care quality a high priority.
- Recognize the importance of team building, leadership, and family centeredness in performing effective CQI.
- Seek opportunities to initiate or actively participate in CQI projects. Work collaboratively to help create and maintain a CQI culture within the institution.
- Model professional behavior when reviewing and interpreting data.

SYSTEMS ORGANIZATION AND IMPROVEMENT

In order to improve efficiency and quality in their organizations, pediatric hospitalists should:
- Engage Hospital Senior Management, Hospital Board of Directors and Medical Staff leadership in creating, implementing, and sustaining short and long term quality improvement goals.
- Participate on Quality Improvement committees and seek opportunities to serve as Quality Improvement Officers or Consultants.
- Advocate for the necessary information systems and other infrastructure to secure accurate data and assure success in the CQI process.

COST-EFFECTIVE CARE

INTRODUCTION

The delivery of cost-effective care is an important responsibility and necessary skill for pediatric hospitalists. In the United States, hospital care for children, including neonatal conditions, pediatric illness and adolescent pregnancy entails 6.3 million hospital stays and $46 billion in charges per year. Pediatric inpatient care accounts for 18% of all hospital days and 9% of total U.S. hospital charges. Of these,, three respiratory conditions - pneumonia, bronchitis and asthma - are responsible for nearly $3 billion in charges or 7% of the total US health care bill for children and adolescents Although some categories of hospital expenses such as nurses or equipment may be outside the control of physicians, there are a number that are driven by physician practice patterns. Physician influence on hospital costs is exerted primarily through hospital length stay, medication prescribing patterns, and utilization of laboratory and diagnostic imaging services. Pediatric hospitalists can make a significant contribution to cost management efforts by increased awareness, standardization, evaluation and modification of practice and utilization patterns.

KNOWLEDGE

Pediatric hospitalists should be able to:
- List the various methods of financing health care for children and state the implications of each on patient care.
- Identify and discuss the importance of the metrics used to describe hospital costs such as charges, length of stay, cost per case, and hospital expense per adjusted day.
- Demonstrate knowledge of common payment mechanisms for hospital care such as case rates, percent of charges, observation status, per diem rates, and capitation.
- Describe mechanisms used by health plans and hospitals to limit hospital costs including pre-authorization and utilization review.
- Name hospital care costs that are controllable by physicians.
- Identify examples of how standardization of clinical care processes improves cost and quality of care.
- Discuss recent trends in health care delivery that affect pediatric practice such as coordinated management of complex chronic diseases and development of integrated delivery systems.
- Describe the concept of system integration and define the roles of various components of the health care system such as community health centers, academic health centers, private practices, and home care agencies.
- Define the role of major federal health programs such as Medicaid, Women Infants and Children (WIC) and Vaccines for Children (VFC) in funding healthcare to children from low-income households.
- Give an example of differences in costs of commonly prescribed medications. Illustrate the importance of various considerations when prescribing drugs such as total cost, compliance, availability of pediatric formulation, and insurance formulary lists.

SKILLS

Pediatric hospitalists should be able to:
- Apply strategies to control costs in the daily care of patients in the hospital, such as use of generic drugs, case management, and avoidance of ordering unnecessary tests, as appropriate.
- Participate in hospital committees where finance and clinical care are discussed such as pharmacy and therapeutics, quality improvement, ambulatory access, and others.
- Incorporate cost considerations when writing orders, and use these opportunities to educate trainees on the importance of such considerations.
- Obtain information about costs of care including drugs, medical imaging, and devices.
- Work with consultants to determine cost effective approaches to testing and treatment plans.
- Coordinate the care of patients to reduce redundant testing or procedures.
- Work effectively with home care, discharge planning nurses, care coordinators, and case managers to ensure timely and safe hospital discharge.
- Provide education for patients and the family/caregiver that promotes an awareness of costs in developing treatment and discharge plans.
- Develop and utilize metrics and performance reporting (such as medication usage) to improve delivery of cost effective care.

ATTITUDES

Pediatric hospitalists should be able to:
- Assume personal responsibility for providing cost effective care.
- Serve as an advocate among professional colleagues and in the community for methods to reduce costs of care.
- Work collaboratively with others to continuously evaluate and improve care while reducing costs.

SYSTEMS ORGANIZATION AND IMPROVEMENT

In order to improve efficiency and quality within their organizations, pediatric hospitalists should:
- Support efforts to gather and disseminate cost, quality and safety data for use in monitoring quality and business improvement efforts.
- Promote standard methods of clinical care that improve cost, quality and patient safety.
- Work to develop benchmarks for "best practices" in cost effective care.
- Collaborate with hospital administrators to determine and direct policies that impact healthcare utilization.

EDUCATION

INTRODUCTION

Pediatric hospitalists can serve many roles in education, from educating hospital staff, trainees (medical students, residents, and fellows), community clinicians and organizations and colleagues, to investing in self-education. Many hospitalists derive their academic identity from their pivotal role in teaching trainees or ancillary staff on the hospital wards and in directing training programs. Training future hospitalists and directing continuing medical education programs to enable current hospitalists to update their knowledge and skills are educational opportunities which are emerging as core competencies for the field are defined. Competencies listed below should be addressed in the context of the specific learner-educator environment.

KNOWLEDGE

Pediatric hospitalists should be able to:
- Discuss how the principles of adult learning theory, such as those listed below, can be used in leading daily learning activities.
    - Assessment of learning needs
    - Case-based approach building on the learner's previous experiences or encounters
    - Reflection
    - Recognition of the "teachable moment"
    - Active learning
    - Provide an effective learning environment
    - Self-directed learning
    - Modeling
    - Establish learning goals
- Describe one's own preferred teaching and learning style and discuss how this may affect learners with different learning styles.
- Identify the steps involved in designing a learning activity, curriculum or program which include:
    - Conduct a needs assessment to determine learner needs
    - Write competency-based goals and objectives based upon learner needs to define what is to be accomplished.
    - Define and secure resources (personnel, readings, handouts, computer programs, and time)
    - Actively involve learners in attaining competencies
    - Evaluate the learners' attainment of competencies
    - Evaluate the effectiveness of the activity, curriculum or program
- Define competencies, performance indicators, goals and objectives, and explain their role in the evaluation of physicians.
- Describe the pediatric competencies currently required by regulatory agencies such as the Accreditation Council for Graduate Medical Education (ACGME) and the American Board of Pediatrics (ABP). Explain why a continuum of competencies throughout a professional career is required, and illustrate the benefits and challenges of this expectation.
- Give illustrative examples of resident performance that fall within each of the six mandated ACGME competency domains: patient care, medical knowledge, practice-based learning and improvement, interpersonal skills and communications, professionalism, and systems-based practice.
- List specific examples of how pediatric hospitalists can educate to each of the six core competencies, attending to the role on the ward and in the larger healthcare system.
- Explain how learners benefit from knowing their learning goals at the start of an educational experience.
- Compare the strengths and weaknesses of the following evaluation methods: oral exams, written tests, global evaluations, direct observations with checklists, and multi-source (360 degree) evaluations.
- Compare and contrast formative feedback with summative evaluation.
- Describe the typical effects of evaluation on the motivation and learning priorities of both medical students and residents.
- Identify how key concepts of evidence-based medicine literature review should be used to create a plan of evaluation and management for patients.
- List resources and activities for continuous learning to maintain current knowledge and skills.

SKILLS

Pediatric hospitalists should be able to:
- Orient trainees to inpatient ward rotation expectations, including learning goals and objectives, patient care and team responsibilities, systems, policies and procedures for the rotation.
- Identify the educational objectives and the learner's educational needs in various settings. Use this information to direct selection of content and teaching methods.
- Demonstrate efficient and flexible use of time when teaching, adapting the mix of teaching and independent learning activities to optimize use of the time available.
- Develop a repertoire of teaching and supervision methods that enhance a learner's knowledge base, clinical skills, and attitudes/behaviors, including:
  - Bedside teaching
  - Teaching during work rounds
  - Lectures or case-based discussions using multimedia presentation methods
  - Teaching a specific skill or procedure
  - Affirm competency when learner masters a skill
  - Role modeling for learners, with articulation of thought process
  - Written instruction
- Provide frequent, effective feedback based upon direct observation of trainee's clinical, communication, and technical skills and professionalism.
- Teach effectively in large group settings, such as hospital or community setting conferences.
- Teach effectively in small groups using a case-based format.
  - Use different types of questioning (broadening, justifying, hypothetical, and alternative)
  - Address learning needs of trainees of different levels of experience
- Teach patients and the family/caregiver about the diagnosis, planned investigation, management plan and prognosis in an interactive, family centered manner.

ATTITUDES

Pediatric hospitalists should be able to:
- Promote a climate of continuous learning by acknowledging one's own knowledge gaps and prompting learners to teach each other.
- Model effective and empathetic communication with patients and the family/caregiver when educating.
- Encourage trainees to be self-directed and to learn independently.
- Model professional behavior by being prompt, prepared, available, and approachable in educational efforts.
- Build and maintain teamwork by providing reinforcing as well as corrective feedback.

SYSTEMS ORGANIZATION AND IMPROVEMENT

In order to improve efficiency and quality within their organizations, pediatric hospitalists should:
- Partner with training programs to create, maintain, and implement inpatient hospital medicine education.
- Work with hospital administrators to maintain adequate trainee supervision to ensure patient safety, while encouraging development of autonomous practice.
- Through educational efforts, promote quality improvement, patient safety, cost effective care, evidence based medicine and effective communication around inpatient pediatric care.
- Integrate and explain the rationale behind established clinical pathways and prompt trainees to use them consistently.
- Address the balance of teaching and patient care responsibilities with hospital administration and training program directors to maximize the effectiveness of both.
- Collaborate with hospital administration to ensure adequate teaching facilities.

ETHICS

INTRODUCTION

Morality is the "right" or "wrong" of human conduct, where ethics is the disciplined study of the justification for rules of human conduct. Morality concerns obligations of what ought to be and what virtues should be cultivated to sustain a truly moral society. The field of bioethics (or medical ethics) applies theory to address ethical issues in medicine, including those that arise during the care of patients as well as those focused on organizations and policy. Bioethics focuses on what morality should be for patients, healthcare professionals, healthcare institutions, and healthcare policy. The rights and responsibilities of patients and the fiduciary responsibility of healthcare providers to patients are central to this definition. Pediatric hospitalists must have a basic knowledge of ethical principles to provide balanced, ethical care.

KNOWLEDGE

Pediatric hospitalists should be able to:

- Describe the core principles of ethics: beneficence, justice, respect for autonomy, and non-maleficence.
- Discuss the four virtues of a fiduciary- self-effacement, self-sacrifice, compassion, and integrity.
- Identify the elements of informed consent and describe the concept of informed assent.
- Describe special circumstances impacting the informed consent process specific to the pediatric population, such as patients in the juvenile justice system, ward of the court, emancipated minors, child protection cases, and others.
- Describe the role and composition of the hospital Ethics Committee.
- Compare and contrast the fiduciary responsibilities of the institution, insurer, and healthcare provider and discuss the impact of these on delivery of ethical patient care.
- Distinguish between substantive justice (concern that the outcomes of a process is fair) and procedural justice (concern that the decision-making process itself is fair).
- Describe how ethical principles can inform development of healthcare policy.
- Give examples of how patients and the family/caregiver meet ethical obligations to healthcare professionals (such as engagement in informed consent), to others in the household (such as discussions on undue burden to other members), and society (such as appropriate allocation of resources).
- Explain the concept of medical futility and its shortcomings.

SKILLS

Pediatric hospitalists should be able to:

- Apply ethical principles to daily patient care.
- Obtain informed consent and assent, as appropriate.
- Access legal support as needed to obtain consent to treat as appropriate in special circumstances.
- Communicate effectively, maintaining confidentiality and patient privacy.
- Identify situations involving ethical conflict, and take steps to resolve this conflict.
- Consult the Ethics Committee/Team appropriately.

ATTITUDES

Pediatric hospitalists should be able to:

- Acknowledge personal biases that impact ethical decision-making.
- Recognize gaps in knowledge and seek opportunities for ethics education.
- Role model ethical practices.

SYSTEMS ORGANIZATION AND IMPROVEMENT

In order to improve efficiency and quality in their organizations, pediatric hospitalists should:

- Work with hospital administration to identify and modify institutional practices and policies to assure ethical healthcare delivery.
- Advocate for healthcare policy that ensures appropriate access to healthcare services for children.

EVIDENCE-BASED MEDICINE

INTRODUCTION

Evidence-based medicine (EBM) is the judicious use of systematically evaluated clinical research applied to care of a patient or population. Evidence-based medicine principles support use of results from rigorously validated randomized controlled trials where available, in combination with other sources of information such as other published literature, expert opinion and consensus statements. Grading research based on a hierarchy of strength of evidence is a hallmark of EBM. Clinical decisions are then made considering a combination of a patient's value system, specific clinical circumstances, and a thorough assessment of the literature regarding the clinical condition. Used correctly, application of EBM results in use of current best scientific knowledge to create best plans of care while acknowledging the specific circumstance of patients.

KNOWLEDGE

Pediatric hospitalists should be able to:
- Define EBM and state how its use is integrated into clinical decision-making for a patient or a population.
- Review how EBM support quality improvement and patient safety efforts.
- List databases and other resources commonly used to search for medical evidence.
- Discuss the risk and benefits of accessing medical resources through publicly available search engines.
- Discuss the benefits and limitations of commonly used scientific medical resources, considering issues such as publication bias, consensus statement methodology used, national versus international web indexed articles, and others.
- Explain the classification systems used to grade the strength of evidence in a given published work and discuss how this can help guide clinical decision making.
- Explain how each of the components (PICO, or patient-intervention-control-outcomes) of a well composed, searchable clinical question aid in obtaining a more accurate and comprehensive list of references.
- Distinguish between different study designs, such as retrospective, prospective, case control, and others and list the benefits and limitations of each.
- Compare and contrast the major study types such as cost-effectiveness, therapy, diagnosis, prognosis, harm, and systematic review.
- Define commonly used terms such as relative and absolute risk reduction, number needed to treat (NNT), sensitivity, specificity, positive and negative predictive values (PPV, NPV), likelihood ratios (LR).

SKILLS

Pediatric hospitalists should be able to:
- Demonstrate facility with internet search engines to access all potentially relevant sources of information.
- Access on line evidence-based medicine toolkits to assist with the assessment of healthcare literature.
- Translate a clinical question into a searchable PICO question or search string.
- Identify the type of clinical question being asked: therapy, diagnosis, prognosis or harm/causality.
- Identify the most appropriate study design for a given specific question.
- Demonstrate proficiency in performance of an EBM literature search using electronic resources such as Pub Med.
- Critically appraise the quality of studies, using a consistent method.
- Critically interpret study results.
- Apply relevant results of validated studies that are of the highest quality available to care for individual patients and populations.
- Develop a personal strategy to consistently incorporate evidence, balance of harm and benefits, and patients' values into clinical decision making to deliver the highest quality care.

ATTITUDES

Pediatric hospitalists should be able to:
- Seek the best available evidence to support clinical decision making.
- Acquire and maintain EBM skills through integration into daily practice and pursuit of ongoing continuing education.
- Recognize how personal practice patterns are influenced by the integration of EBM.
- Role model use of EBM at the beside.

SYSTEMS ORGANIZATION AND IMPROVEMENT

In order to improve efficiency and quality within their organizations, pediatric hospitalists should:

- Lead, coordinate or participate in the development and implementation cost-effective, evidence-based care pathways to standardize the evaluation and management of hospitalized children in the local system.
- Engage with hospital staff, subspecialists, and others in a multidisciplinary team approach toward integrating EBM into clinical decision making processes.
- Work with hospital administrators to acquire and maintain effective, efficient electronic resources for the performance of EBM.

HEALTH INFORMATION SYSTEMS

INTRODUCTION

Health information systems encompass the range of technology in health care used to acquire, store, deliver and analyze medical data. In the hospital environment, this technology is one of the most important components to the delivery of high-quality and safe care. In particular, healthcare provider order entry, has been shown to reduce medical errors, while systems that display recently completed laboratory testing may decrease redundant testing. Despite these benefits, hospitals have been slow to adopt these technologies. The Institute of Medicine and the Department of Health and Human Services have recognized this fact and have begun serious efforts to improve the adoption of electronic medical information systems in all health care environments. Pediatric hospitalists use these systems for clinical care, education, quality improvement efforts and research and can assist with assessing and implementing systems

KNOWLEDGE

Pediatric hospitalists should be able to:

- Compare and contrast the varied health information systems used to manage medical information across different hospital settings, especially with regard to the differences between adult and pediatric needs.
- Describe the importance of proper storage and retrieval of protected health information.
- Discuss the impact of the Health Insurance Portability and Accountability Act of 1996 (HIPAA) Privacy Rule on health information systems security.
- Explain the value of clinical decision support in rendering patient care.
- Compare and contrast the influence of electronic health information on practice management, clinical decision-making, quality improvement projects and performance of research.
- Identify at least one improvement in patient safety that can be realized with institution of an electronic medical record.
- Describe how hospital policies and procedures impact information systems operations, and that in turn delivery of health care to children influences these policies, procedures, and systems.
- Describe the basic organization of the information technology department.
- Describe resources that can be accessed to address questions about information systems such as a hospital "HELP" desk, vendor support lines, or online access to other healthcare providers who use the system.
- Delineate how staff dedicated to information technology support quality and safety efforts and data retrieval.
- List information resources and tools available to support life-long learning.
- Discuss the importance of pediatric hospitalists in creating, modifying, and evaluating changes to health information systems.
- Describe the unique needs of children in regard to information technology, and the importance of careful design and implementation of health information systems in hospitals and clinics that care for children.

SKILLS

Pediatric hospitalists should be able to:

- Demonstrate proficiency with foundational computer skills (email, literature searching, downloading and uploading files.) and common computer applications (word processing, spreadsheet use, and presentation software) as well as the local provider order entry system.
- Skillfully access and use web-based educational resources for continuing education and enrichment of trainee learning experiences.
- Effectively and efficiently utilize local health information systems for clinical care, education, and performance of projects as appropriate within the context of the local system.

- Assist in creation of order sets and documentation templates.
- Assess the value of rules and alerts and assist with editing these as appropriate.

ATTITUDES

Pediatric hospitalists should be able to:
- Be accountable for working to ensure the successful functioning of health information systems.
- Advocate for the proper alignment of health information systems choices with clinical needs.
- Effectively communicate with information systems managers.
- Respect patient confidentiality by using the security-directed features of information systems.

SYSTEMS ORGANIZATION AND IMPROVEMENT

In order to improve efficiency and quality within their organizations, pediatric hospitalists should:
- Participate in appropriate hospital committees and assist with information technology solutions to address causes of unsafe care.
- Work with hospital administrators and the Medical Staff to integrate new technologies to the practice of medicine (such as telemedicine, medical decision making, computerized medical records, electronic information networks and others).
- Seek opportunities to improve the role of information technology in managing costs, quality improvement efforts, and research, if applicable.

LEGAL ISSUES / RISK MANAGEMENT

INTRODUCTION

Risk Management is a discipline commonly perceived to be the domain of the institutional personnel and committees who are called upon to administer the aftermath of adverse events. However, consequence management is far from the most effective utilization of such resources, as they are most efficiently and ethically deployed in preventive programs. Risk management therefore prospectively draws upon the disciplines of law, patient safety, quality improvement, systems management, ethics, and human resources in addition to medicine, in an effort to eliminate or ameliorate the undesirable consequences of delivering healthcare services.

KNOWLEDGE

Pediatric hospitalists should be able to:
- Summarize the regulatory and legal stipulations that may impact pediatric hospitalists' contracting and practice including:
  - Anti-kickback regulations (Stark Rules)
  - Anti-trust regulations (Sherman Act)
  - Billing rules, coding for services, collections (Fraud and Abuse regulations)
  - Transfer / transport of patients (Emergency Medical Treatment and Active Labor Act (EMTALA))
  - Utilization review and managed care issues
- Describe the behavioral and physical characteristics of the impaired practitioner, including fatigue, substance abuse, and disruptive behavior.
- Identify the role of behavior and attitudes in generating patient and family/caregiver complaints.
- Explain the role of formal intervention programs for impaired practitioners.
- State the responsibilities of state medical licensing boards and the Drug Enforcement Agency.
- Summarize the role of the Hospital Medical Staff in granting clinical privileges and initiating disciplinary actions.
- Define the role of the National Practitioner Data Bank.
- List responsibilities associated with maintaining malpractice insurance, including documentation and disclosure requirements).
- Explain the legal definition of negligence.
- Define the terms "assent" and "consent," and describe the circumstances in which informed assent or consent is needed.

- Explain the role of the Health Insurance Portability and Accountability Act of 1996 (HIPAA) Privacy Rule in maintaining patient confidentiality.
- Compare and contrast the malpractice risk in healthcare environments with and without trainees.
- Give an example of legal issues which can arise in various clinical scenarios such as end of life care, "no code" discussions (do-not-resuscitate or allow-natural-death) organ donation, guardianship, and newborn resuscitation.
- Describe the role of pediatric hospitalists in recognizing and reporting family violence (child, spouse and elder abuse).

SKILLS

Pediatric hospitalists should be able to:
- Obtain informed assent and/or consent from patients and/or the family/caregiver.
- Disclose medical errors clearly, concisely and completely to patients and the family/caregiver.
- Accurately communicate in difficult situations and when delivering sensitive information, with compassion and a professional attitude.
- Effectively support and communicate end-of-life decisions and planning.
- Consistently practice patient and family centered care by educating and empowering patients and the family/caregiver thereby enhancing safe delivery of healthcare.
- Transfer patient information concisely and precisely to other healthcare providers during all transitions of care.
- Prescribe treatments safely, using safe medication prescribing practices.
- Consistently document in the medical record with accuracy and appropriate detail.

ATTITUDES

Pediatric hospitalists should be able to:
- Role model professional behavior.
- Respond to complaints in a compassionate and sensitive manner.
- Seek opportunities to learn and practice risk reduction strategies (such as failure modes and effects analysis (FMEA) and others).
- Engage trainees in discussions on the importance of communication and documentation.

SYSTEMS ORGANIZATION AND IMPROVEMENT

In order to improve efficiency and quality within their organizations, pediatric hospitalists should:
- Engage in organizational risk management efforts, and promote risk prevention by active participation in appropriate hospital committees.
- Advocate for healthcare information systems that enhance ease and accuracy of documentation and prescribing.
- Encourage and support efforts to create a comprehensive risk reduction program encompassing education for hospital staff, medical staff, and trainees.

PATIENT SAFETY

INTRODUCTION

The topic of Patient Safety became a major priority for healthcare providers in 1999 when the Institute of Medicine (IOM) report entitled "To Err is Human" focused attention on patient safety and medical errors. The Institute of Medicine defined safety as "freedom from accidental injury" and error as the "failure of a planned action to be completed as intended or the use of a wrong plan to achieve an aim". The IOM report estimated that between 44,000 to 98,000 Americans die each year as a result of medical errors which exceed the number attributable to the 8th leading cause of death in America. Total national costs of preventable adverse events are estimated to be up to $29 billion. Since the initial publication of the 1999 IOM report, there have been a number of local, state, and national programs focused on reducing error. Efforts over the past few years have attempted to better classify errors by the harm caused, allowing targeted interventions to specifically address these more clinically significant events. Children, as a vulnerable population, are at particular risk for medical errors and specifically medication errors.

Pediatric hospitalists have an exceptional opportunity to promote patient safety and help develop systems that will reduce harm in the inpatient arena.

KNOWLEDGE

Pediatric hospitalists should be able to:
- Identify the basic principles of patient safety as outlined in the original 1999 IOM report.
- Describe the culture necessary for successful safety efforts. Define "Just" culture.
- Define commonly used terms and tools of Patient Safety such as reliability, transparency, adverse medical event, harm, preventable errors, failure mode effects analysis (FMEA), root cause analysis (RCA) and trigger tool.
- Name common patient safety practices and enhancements including pre-printed order sets, practice guidelines, electronic health information systems, bar coding, time-outs, and others. Explain how new errors can be associated with the introduction of these enhancements.
- Discuss why errors are more often a result of systems failures rather than individual failures.
- Explain how decreasing unwanted variability in care impacts patient safety.
- Illustrate that building safety into everyday processes of care is the most effective way to reduce or prevent errors.
- Describe how patient safety is threatened by poor information transfer and failed communication.
- Discuss strategies for effective, efficient, and safe communications that impact all aspects of patient care such as handoffs between healthcare providers, team rounds, family engagement, and others. List the strengths and limitations of different communication methods.
- Describe the effects of sleep quality and quantity on healthcare providers and the impact on patient safety.
- Summarize the components of family centered care and discuss the importance of engaging patients and the family/caregiver in safety efforts.
- Define the role of the Joint Commission (TJC) in hospital accreditation and describe how pediatric hospitalists can help assure relevant standards are met.
- Articulate TJC guidelines on patient safety and the National Patient Safety Goals.
- Discuss factors unique to children that lead to increased risk for medication errors, attending to weight-based dosing, developmental physiology, compounding and drug delivery methods, and others.
- Discuss how financial reimbursement from private and government payers can be tied to preventable patient safety events.
- List the common national societies and agencies [such as the Institute for Healthcare Improvement (IHI), American Academy of Pediatrics (AAP), TJC, Centers for Medicare and Medicaid Services (CMS)] influencing inpatient pediatric safety measures and describe pediatric hospitalists' role in responding to their statements.
- Delineate the role of pediatric hospitalists in assuring proper supervision of trainees and the impact of this on patient safety.

SKILLS

Pediatric hospitalists should be able to:
- Arrange safe and efficient hospital admissions and discharges, addressing issues such as level of nursing care needed and coordination of care, respectively.
- Proactively identify sources of potential patient harm, including environmental and personal factors that affect your ability to render safe medical care. Develop a plan to address appropriate negative influences.
- Consistently adhere to patient safety principles when providing direct patient care such as when ordering treatment, performing procedures, and communicating care plans.
- Set performance standards and expectations for patient safety in the hospital setting.
- Educate trainees, nursing staff, ancillary staff and peers on basic safety principles.
- Demonstrate proficiency in using the institution's safety reporting system.
- Work effectively and collaboratively with safety teams, utilizing safety tools including reduction of process complexity, building in redundancy, improving team functioning and identifying team members' assumptions.
- Implement and serve as a physician champion for patient safety initiatives that protect children from harm.
- Actively contribute during ad hoc and sentinel event reviews.
- Disclose medical errors clearly, concisely and completely to patients and/or caregivers.

ATTITUDES

Pediatric hospitalists should be able to:
- Seek opportunities to be involved in strategies to eliminate harm.
- Role model effective infection control practices in daily patient care activities.
- Build an awareness of the need for and will for change to make patient safety a high and consistent priority.
- Model behavior and take initiative in reporting medical errors.
- Work collaboratively to help create an open culture of safety within the institution.

SYSTEMS ORGANIZATION AND IMPROVEMENT

In order to improve efficiency and quality within their organizations, pediatric hospitalists should:
- Engage the hospital senior management, the hospital board of directors and the medical staff leadership in making patient safety one of the top strategic priorities for the institution.
- Advocate for the necessary information systems and other infrastructure to secure accurate data and assure success with safety initiatives.
- Participate on patient safety committees at the group or systems level and seek opportunities to serve as medical safety officers or medical safety consultants locally or nationally.

RESEARCH

INTRODUCTION

Research is a rapidly growing aspect of inpatient medicine. The practice of evidence-based medicine and the acute need for more evidence on inpatient conditions require that pediatric hospitalists understand and participate in research related activities. Pediatric hospitalists' role in research will vary depending on their setting and job description. This role may include many facets, from reviewing relevant patient-based articles, to participating in multi-institutional studies requiring enrollment of patients, to leading local or national studies. Pediatric hospitalists need to have a basic understanding of research methods and process in order to participate in and benefit from research. This understanding contributes to the effective care of hospitalized patients.

KNOWLEDGE

Pediatric hospitalists should be able to:
- Compare and contrast different types of study design such as case-control, cohort, observational, and randomized control trials. Understand the advantages and disadvantages of each study design.
- Name resources available to access current or proposed studies and funding sources such as the Agency for Healthcare Research and Quality (AHRQ), the National Institutes of Health (NIH), Robert Wood Johnson Foundation, clinicaltrials.gov, and others.
- Discuss what resources are required to support research components of data collection, data analysis, abstract and manuscript preparation, grant funding and others.
- Explain how results from articles published in the following formats apply to clinical practice:
  - Case reports and case series
  - Retrospective chart reviews
  - Secondary data analyses of large data sets
  - Randomized controlled trials
  - Meta analyses and systematic reviews
  - Practice Guidelines
- Identify and efficiently locate the best available information resources to address questions in clinical practice, and conduct computerized scientific literature searches in a planned and systematic fashion.
- Define basic statistical terms such as sample, discrete and continuous data variables, measures of central tendency (mean, median, and mode) and variability (variance, standard deviation, range).
- Cite the various aspects of the research process including informed consent or assent, the role of institutional review boards (IRB), and HIPAA (Health Insurance Portability and Accountability Act).
- Discuss special protections needed when conducting research with vulnerable populations. Define "minimal risk" for a healthy child and for a child with an illness.

- List common barriers to implementation of clinical studies and describe pediatric hospitalists' role in overcoming these barriers.

SKILLS

Pediatric hospitalists should be able to:
- Demonstrate proficiency in searching the medical literature for existing relevant clinical research for their inpatients.
- Generate an answerable patient-centered clinical question that is relevant to improving patient care.
- Apply the results of studies to clinical practice by determining whether the study subjects were similar to patients being treated, whether all clinically important outcomes were considered, identify threats to validity, and
  - For treatment studies, describe whether the likely benefits are worth the potential harm and cost.
  - For studies of diagnostic tests, describe whether the test is available, affordable, accurate and precise in the present clinical setting, and whether the results of the test will change the management of patients being treated.
  - For studies of harm, describe whether the magnitude of risk warrants an attempt to stop the exposure.
  - For studies of prognosis, describe whether the results of the study will lead directly to selecting therapy and/or are useful for counseling patients.
- Provide effective informed consent or assent for patients participating in research studies as appropriate.

ATTITUDES

Pediatric hospitalists should be able to:
- Appreciate the importance of full informed consent for purposes of patient participation in clinical research.
- Appreciate the importance of patient assent, even in the presence of legal guardian informed consent, when involving children in clinical research.
- Demonstrate highly ethical principles in participating in research studies.
- Avoid conflict of interest or potential conflict of interest in participation in research studies.
- Acquire, manage, and share data collected for research purposes in a responsible and professional manner, maintaining high standards for protecting confidentiality, avoiding unjustified exclusions, sharing data, and adhering to copyright law.

SYSTEMS ORGANIZATION AND IMPROVEMENT

In order to improve efficiency and quality within their organizations, pediatric hospitalists should:
- Encourage participation of interdisciplinary teams including nursing, social work, nutrition, pharmacy, and others in performance of research.
- Advocate for thoughtful application of research findings to improve systems of healthcare delivery.
- Support national multi-center research efforts that improve the evidence base in inpatient pediatrics. Where appropriate, encourage participation local hospital involvement in these efforts.
- Recognize, support and promote efforts of research team members (analyst, data collector, statistician, nursing, and others).

TRANSITIONS OF CARE

INTRODUCTION

Transitions of care occur when a patient moves from one level of care to another or from one institution to another. One component of transitions of care is the patient handoff, which refers to the interaction between providers when responsibility for patient care is transferred from one provider to another. Ineffective transitions of care jeopardize patient safety and may result in adverse events, increased healthcare utilization, and patient or caregiver stress. Thus, every transition of care should involve a set of actions designed to ensure that the transfer is safe, efficient, and effective. Pediatric hospitalists are routinely involved in patient transfers and can lead institutional efforts to promote optimal patient handoffs and transitions of care.

KNOWLEDGE

Pediatric hospitalists should be able to:

- Compare and contrast patient handoffs with transitions of care.
- List the critical elements that should be communicated between providers at the time of a patient handoff, and describe how these elements may vary depending on characteristics of the patient or the provider.
- List the relevant information that should be communicated during each transition of care to ensure patient safety and promote the continuum of care.
- Explain the pros and cons of different modes of communication in the context of the various types of patient transfers.
- Differentiate between the available levels of care and determine the most appropriate option for each patient, taking the need for isolation and level of nursing care into account.
- Describe the impact of the Emergency Medical Treatment and Active Labor Act (EMTALA) on patient transfers.
- Articulate the National Patient Safety Goals that relate to transitions of care, including effectiveness of communication and medication reconciliation.

SKILLS

Pediatric hospitalists should be able to:

- Prepare concise clinical summaries in preparation for patient handoffs or transitions of care, incorporating key elements as appropriate.
- Utilize the most efficient and reliable mode of communication for each transition of care.
- Arrange safe and efficient transfers to, from, and within the inpatient setting.
- Promptly review the medical information received from referring providers and clarify any discrepancies when accepting a new patient.
- Anticipate needs at the time of discharge and begin discharge planning early in the hospitalization.
- Provide legible and clear discharge instructions that take into account the primary language and reading level of the patient and caregiver and include information about available resources after discharge should questions arise.
- Communicate effectively with the primary care provider and other providers as necessary at the time of admission, discharge, and when there is a significant change in clinical status.
- Accurately and completely reconcile medications during transitions of care.
- Develop systems to ensure the future comprehensive review of patient data that was pending at the time of discharge.

ATTITUDES

Pediatric hospitalists should be able to:

- Appreciate the impact of ineffective handoffs and transitions of care on patient safety and quality of care.
- Demonstrate respect for referring physicians and seek their input when developing protocols for communication during transitions of care.
- Appreciate the impact of the transfer on the patient and caregiver and ensure their goals and preferences are incorporated into the care plan at all stages of the transition of care.
- Take responsibility for the coordination of a multidisciplinary approach to patient and caregiver education in preparation for the transition of care.
- Maintain availability to patients, caregivers, and providers after transitions of care should questions arise.

SYSTEMS ORGANIZATION AND IMPROVEMENT

Pediatric hospitalists should be able to:

- Lead, coordinate, or participate in the ongoing evaluation and improvement of the referral, admission, and discharge processes at their institution, taking into account input from stakeholders.
- Lead, coordinate, or participate in initiatives to develop and implement systems that promote timely and effective communication between providers during handoffs and transitions of care.

Pediatric Hospital Medicine Core Competencies: Development and Methodology

Erin R. Stucky, MD[1]
Mary C. Ottolini, MD, MPH[2]
Jennifer Maniscalco, MD, MPH[3]

[1] Rady Children's Hospital San Diego and University of California San Diego School of Medicine Department of Pediatrics.

[2] Children's National Medical Center and the George Washington University School of Medicine Department of Pediatrics.

[3] Children's Hospital Los Angeles and the University of Southern California Keck School of Medicine Department of Pediatrics.

Background: Pediatric hospital medicine is the most rapidly growing site-based pediatric specialty. There are over 2500 unique members in the three core societies in which pediatric hospitalists are members: the American Academy of Pediatrics (AAP), the Academic Pediatric Association (APA) and the Society of Hospital Medicine (SHM). Pediatric hospitalists are fulfilling both clinical and system improvement roles within varied hospital systems. Defined expectations and competencies for pediatric hospitalists are needed.

Methods: In 2005, SHM's Pediatric Core Curriculum Task Force initiated the project and formed the editorial board. Over the subsequent four years, multiple pediatric hospitalists belonging to the AAP, APA, or SHM contributed to the content of and guided the development of the project. Editors and collaborators created a framework for identifying appropriate competency content areas. Content experts from both within and outside of pediatric hospital medicine participated as contributors. A number of selected national organizations and societies provided valuable feedback on chapters. The final product was validated by formal review from the AAP, APA, and SHM.

Results: The *Pediatric Hospital Medicine Core Competencies* were created. They include 54 chapters divided into four sections: Common Clinical Diagnoses and Conditions, Core Skills, Specialized Clinical Services, and Healthcare Systems: Supporting and Advancing Child Health. Each chapter can be used independently of the others. Chapters follow the knowledge, skills, and attitudes educational curriculum format, and have an additional section on systems organization and improvement to reflect the pediatric hospitalist's responsibility to advance systems of care.

Conclusion: These competencies provide a foundation for the creation of pediatric hospital medicine curricula and serve to standardize and improve inpatient training practices. *Journal of Hospital Medicine* 2010;5(4)(Suppl 2):82–86. © 2010 Society of Hospital Medicine.

KEYWORDS: hospitalist, hospital medicine, pediatric, child, competency, curriculum, methodology.

Introduction

The Society of Hospital Medicine (SHM) defines hospitalists as physicians whose primary professional focus is the comprehensive general medical care of hospitalized patients. Their activities include patient care, teaching, research, and leadership related to Hospital Medicine.[1] It is estimated that there are up to 2500 pediatric hospitalists in the United States, with continued growth due to the converging needs for a dedicated focus on patient safety, quality improvement, hospital throughput, and inpatient teaching.[2-9] (Pediatric Hospital Medicine (PHM), as defined today, has been practiced in the United States for at least 30 years[10] and continues to evolve as an area of specialization, with the refinement of a distinct knowledgebase and skill set focused on the provision of high quality general pediatric care in the inpatient setting. PHM is the latest site-specific specialty to emerge from the field of general pediatrics – it's development analogous to the evolution of critical care or emergency medicine during previous decades.[11] Adult hospital medicine has defined itself within the field of general internal medicine[12] and has recently received approval to provide a recognized focus of practice exam in 2010 for those re-certifying with the American Board of Internal Medicine,[13] PHM is creating an identity as a subspecialty practice with distinct focus on inpatient care for children within the larger context of general pediatric care.[8,14]

The *Pediatric Hospital Medicine Core Competencies* were created to help define the roles and expectations for pediatric hospitalists, regardless of practice setting. The intent is to provide a unified approach toward identifying the specific body of knowledge and measurable skills needed to assure delivery of the highest quality of care for all hospitalized pediatric patients. Most children requiring hospitalization in the United States are hospitalized in community settings where subspecialty support is more limited and many pediatric services may be unavailable. Children with complex, chronic medical problems, however, are more likely to be hospitalized at a tertiary care or academic institutions. In

2010 Society of Hospital Medicine DOI 10.1002/jhm.774
Published online in wiley InterScience (www.interscience.wiley.com).

order to unify pediatric hospitalists who work in different practice environments, the *PHM Core Competencies* were constructed to represent the knowledge, skills, attitudes, and systems improvements that all pediatric hospitalists can be expected to acquire and maintain.

Furthermore, the content of the *PHM Core Competencies* reflect the fact that children are a vulnerable population. Their care requires attention to many elements which distinguishes it from that given to the majority of the adult population: dependency, differences in developmental physiology and behavior, occurrence of congenital genetic disorders and age-based clinical conditions, impact of chronic disease states on whole child development, and weight-based medication dosing often with limited guidance from pediatric studies, to name a few. Awareness of these needs must be heightened when a child enters the hospital where diagnoses, procedures, and treatments often include use of high-risk modalities and require coordination of care across multiple providers.

Pediatric hospitalists commonly work to improve the systems of care in which they operate and therefore both clinical and non-clinical topics are included. The 54 chapters address the fundamental and most common components of inpatient care but are not an extensive review of all aspects of inpatient medicine encountered by those caring for hospitalized children. Finally, the *PHM Core Competencies* are not intended for use in assessing proficiency immediately post-residency, but do provide a framework for the education and evaluation of both physicians-in-training and practicing hospitalists. Meeting these competencies is anticipated to take from one to three years of active practice in pediatric hospital medicine, and may be reached through a combination of practice experience, course work, self-directed work, and/or formalized training.

Methods

Timeline

In 2002, SHM convened an educational summit from which there was a resolution to create core competencies. Following the summit, the SHM Pediatric Core Curriculum Task Force (CCTF) was created, which included 12 pediatric hospitalists practicing in academic and community facilities, as well as teaching and non-teaching settings, and occupying leadership positions within institutions of varied size and geographic location. Shortly thereafter, in November 2003, approximately 130 pediatric hospitalists attended the first PHM meeting in San Antonio, Texas.[11] At this meeting, with support from leaders in pediatric emergency medicine, first discussions regarding PHM scope of practice were held.

Formal development of the competencies began in 2005 in parallel to but distinct from SHM's adult work, which culminated in *The Core Competencies in Hospital Medicine: A Framework for Curriculum Development* published in 2006. The CCTF divided into three groups, focused on clinical, procedural, and systems-based topics. Face-to-face meetings

TABLE 1. Timeline: Creation of the PHM Core Competencies

Date	Event
Feb 2002	SHM Educational Summit held and CCTF created
Oct 2003	1st PHM meeting held in San Antonio
2003-2007	Chapter focus determined; contributors engaged
2007-2008	APA PHM Special Interest Group (SIG) review; creation of separate PHM Fellowship Competencies (not in this document)
Aug 2008-Oct 2008	SHM Pediatric Committee and CCTF members resume work; editorial review
Oct 2008-Mar 2009	*Internal review*: PHM Fellowship Director, AAP, APA, and SHM section/committee leader, and key national PHM leader reviews solicited and returned
Mar 2009	PHM Fellowship Director comments addressed; editorial review
Mar-Apr 2009	*External reviewers* solicited from national agencies and societies relevant to PHM
Apr-July 2009	External reviewer comments returned
July-Oct 2009	Contributor review of all comments; editorial review, sections revised
Oct 2009	*Final review*: Chapters to SHM subcommittees and Board

were held at the SHM annual meetings, with most work being completed by phone and electronically in the interim periods. In 2007, due to the overlapping interests of the three core pediatric societies, the work was transferred to leaders within the APA. In 2008 the work was transferred back to the leadership within SHM. Since that time, external reviewers were solicited, new chapters created, sections realigned, internal and external reviewer comments incorporated, and final edits for taxonomy, content, and formatting were completed (Table 1).

T1

Areas of Focused Practice

The *PHM Core Competencies* were conceptualized similarly to the SHM adult core competencies. Initial sections were divided into clinical conditions, procedures, and systems. However as content developed and reviewer comments were addressed, the four final sections were modified to those noted in Table 2. For the *Common Clinical Diagnoses and Conditions*, the goal was to select conditions most commonly encountered by pediatric hospitalists. Non-surgical diagnosis-related group (DRG) conditions were selected from the following sources: The Joint Commission's (TJC) Oryx Performance Measures Report[15-16] (asthma, abdominal pain, acute gastroenteritis, simple pneumonia); Child Health Corporation of America's Pediatric Health Information System Dataset (CHCA PHIS, Shawnee Mission, KS), and relevant publications on common pediatric hospitalizations.[17] These data were compared to billing data from randomly-selected practicing hospitalists representing free-standing children's and community hospitals, teaching and non-teaching settings, and urban and rural locations. The 22

T2

2010 Society of Hospital Medicine DOI 10.1002/jhm.774
Published online in wiley InterScience (www.interscience.wiley.com).

TABLE 2. PHM Core Competency Chapters and Sections

Common Clinical Diagnoses and Conditions		Specialized Clinical Services	Core Skills	Healthcare Systems: Supporting and Advancing Child Health
Acute abdominal pain and the acute abdomen	Neonatal fever	Child abuse and neglect	Bladder catheterization/ suprapubic bladder tap	Advocacy
Apparent life-threatening event	Neonatal Jaundice	Hospice and palliative care	Electrocardiogram interpretation	Business practices
Asthma	Pneumonia	Leading a healthcare team	Feeding Tubes	Communication
Bone and joint infections	Respiratory Failure	Newborn care and delivery room management	Fluids and Electrolyte Management	Continuous quality improvement
Bronchiolitis	Seizures	Technology dependent children	Intravenous access and phlebotomy	Cost-effective care
Central nervous system infections	Shock	Transport of the critically ill child	Lumbar puncture	Education
Diabetes mellitus	Sickle cell disease		Non-invasive monitoring	Ethics
Failure to thrive	Skin and soft tissue infection		Nutrition	Evidence based medicine
Fever of unknown origin	Toxic ingestion		Oxygen delivery and airway management	Health Information Systems
Gastroenteritis	Upper airway infections		Pain management	Legal issues/risk management
Kawasaki disease	Urinary Tract infections		Pediatric Advanced Life Support	Patient safety

clinical conditions chosen by the CCTF were those most relevant to the practice of pediatric hospital medicine.

The *Specialized Clinical Services* section addresses important components of care that are not DRG-based and reflect the unique needs of hospitalized children, as assessed by the CCTF, editors, and contributors. *Core Skills* were chosen based on the HCUP Factbook 2 – Procedures,[18] billing data from randomly-selected practicing hospitalists representing the same settings listed above, and critical input from reviewers. Depending on the individual setting, pediatric hospitalists may require skills in areas not found in these 11 chapters, such as chest tube placement or ventilator management. The list is therefore not exhaustive, but rather representative of skills most pediatric hospitalists should maintain.

The *Healthcare Systems: Supporting and Advancing Child Health* chapters are likely the most dissimilar to any core content taught in traditional residency programs. While residency graduates are versed in some components listed in these chapters, comprehensive education in most of these competencies is currently lacking. Improvement of healthcare systems is an essential element of pediatric hospital medicine, and unifies all pediatric hospitalists regardless of practice environment or patient population. Therefore, this section includes chapters that not only focus on systems of care, but also on advancing child health through advocacy, research, education, evidence-based medicine, and ethical practice. These chapters were drawn from a combination of several sources: expectations of external agencies (TJC, Center for Medicaid and Medicare) related to the specific non-clinical work in which pediatric hospitalists are integrally involved; expectations for advocacy as best defined by the AAP and the National Association of Children's Hospitals and Related Institutions (NACHRI); the six core competency domains mandated by the Accrediting Council on Graduate

Medical Education (ACGME), the American Board of Pediatrics (ABP), and hospital medical staff offices as part of Focused Professional Practice Evaluation (FPPE) and Ongoing Professional Practice Evaluation (OPPE)[16]; and assessment of responsibilities and leadership roles fulfilled by pediatric hospitalists in all venues. In keeping with the intent of the competencies to be "timeless", the competency elements call out the need to attend to the changing goals of these groups as well as those of the Institute of Healthcare Improvement (IHI), the Alliance for Pediatric Quality (which consists of ABP, AAP, TJC, CHCA, NACHRI), and local hospital systems leaders.

Contributors and Review

The CCTF selected section (associate) editors from SHM based on established expertise in each area, with input from the SHM Pediatric and Education Committees and the SHM Board. As a collaborative effort, authors for various chapters were solicited in consultation with experts from the AAP, APA, and SHM, and included non-hospitalists with reputations as experts in various fields. Numerous SHM Pediatric Committee and CCTF conference calls were held to review hospital and academic appointments, presentations given, and affiliations relevant to the practice of pediatric hospital medicine. This vetting process resulted in a robust author list representing diverse geographic and practice settings. Contributors were provided with structure (Knowledge, Skills, Attitudes, and Systems subsections) and content (timeless, competency based) guidelines.

The review process was rigorous, and included both internal and external reviewers. The APA review in 2007 included the PHM Special Interest Group as well as the PHM Fellowship Directors (Table 1). After return to SHM and further editing, the internal review commenced which focused on content and scope. The editors addressed the

2010 Society of Hospital Medicine   DOI 10.1002/jhm.774
Published online in wiley InterScience (www.interscience.wiley.com).

resulting suggestions and worked to standardize formatting and use of Bloom's taxonomy.[19] A list of common terms and phrases were created to add consistency between chapters. External reviewers were first mailed a letter requesting interest, which was followed up by emails, letters, and phone calls to encourage feedback. External review included 29 solicited agencies and societies (Table 3), with overall response rate of 66% (41% for Groups I and II). Individual contributors then reviewed comments specific to their chapters, with associate editor overview of their respective sections. The editors reviewed each chapter individually multiple times throughout the 2007-2009 years, contacting individual contributors and reviewers by email and phone. Editors concluded a final comprehensive review of all chapters in late 2009.

Chapter Content

Each of the 54 chapters within the four sections of these competencies is presented in the educational theory of learning domains: Knowledge, Skills, Attitudes, with a final Systems domain added to reflect the emphasis of hospitalist practice on improving healthcare systems. Each chapter is designed to stand alone, which may assist with development of curriculum at individual practice locations. Certain key phrases are apparent throughout, such as "lead, coordinate, or participate in…" and "work with hospital and community leaders to…" which were designed to note the varied roles in different practice settings. Some chapters specifically comment on the application of competency bullets given the unique and differing roles and expectations of pediatric hospitalists, such as research and education. Chapters state specific proficiencies expected wherever possible, with phrases and wording selected to help guide learning activities to achieve the competency.

Application and Future Directions

Although pediatric hospitalists care for children in many settings, these core competencies address the common expectations for any venue. Pediatric hospital medicine requires skills in acute care clinical medicine that attend to the changing needs of hospitalized children. The core of pediatric hospital medicine is dedicated to the care of children in the geographic hospital environment between emergency medicine and tertiary pediatric and neonatal intensive care units. Pediatric hospitalists provide care in related clinical service programs that are linked to hospital systems. In performing these activities, pediatric hospitalists consistently partner with ambulatory providers and subspecialists to render coordinated care across the continuum for a given child. Pediatric hospital medicine is an interdisciplinary practice, with focus on processes of care and clinical quality outcomes based in evidence. Engagement in local, state, and national initiatives to improve child health outcomes is a cornerstone of pediatric hospitalists' practice. These competencies provide the framework for creation of curricula that can reflect local issues and react to changing evidence.

TABLE 3. Solicited Internal and External Reviewers

I. Academic and Certifying Societies
 Academic Pediatric Association
 Accreditation Council for Graduate Medical Education, Pediatric Residency Review
  Committee
 American Academy of Family Physicians
 American Academy of Pediatrics – Board
 American Academy of Pediatrics – National Committee on Hospital Care
 American Association of Critical Care Nursing
 American Board of Family Medicine
 American Board of Pediatrics
 American College of Emergency Physicians
 American Pediatric Society
 Association of American Medical Colleges
 Association of Medical School Pediatric Department Chairs (AMSPDC)
 Association of Pediatric Program Directors
 Council on Teaching Hospitals
 Society of Pediatric Research

II. Stakeholder agencies
 Agency for Healthcare Research and Quality
 American Association of Critical Care Nursing
 American College of Emergency Physicians
 American Hospital Association (AHA)
 American Nurses Association
 American Society of Health-System Pharmacists
 Child Health Corporation of America (CHCA)
 Institute for Healthcare Improvement
 National Association for Children's Hospitals and Related Institutions (NACHRI)
 National Association of Pediatric Nurse Practitioners (NAPNAP)
 National Initiative for Children's Healthcare Quality (NICHQ)
 National Quality Forum
 Quality Resources International
 Robert Wood Johnson Foundation
 The Joint Commission for Accreditation of Hospitals and Organizations (TJC)

III. Pediatric Hospital Medicine Fellowship Directors
 Boston Children's
 Children's Hospital Los Angeles
 Children's National D.C.
 Emory
 Hospital for Sick Kids Toronto
 Rady Children's San Diego – University of California San Diego
 Riley Children's Hospital Indiana
 University of South Florida, All Children's Hospital
 Texas Children's Hospital, Baylor College of Medicine

IV. SHM, APA, AAP Leadership and committee chairs
 American Academy of Pediatrics – Section on Hospital Medicine
 Academic Pediatric Association – PHM Special Interest Group
 SHM Board
 SHM Education Committee
 SHM Family Practice Committee
 SHM Hospital Quality and Patient Safety Committee
 SHM IT Task Force
 SHM Journal Editorial Board
 SHM Palliative Care Task Force
 SHM Practice Analysis Committee
 SHM Public Policy Committee
 SHM Research Committee

As providers of systems-based care, pediatric hospitalists are called upon more and more to render care and provide leadership in clinical arenas that are integral to healthcare organizations, such as home health care, sub-acute care

2010 Society of Hospital Medicine DOI 10.1002/jhm.774
Published online in wiley InterScience (www.interscience.wiley.com).

facilities, and hospice and palliative care programs. The practice of pediatric hospital medicine has evolved to its current state through efforts of many represented in the competencies as contributors, associate editors, editors, and reviewers. Pediatric hospitalists are committed to leading change in healthcare for hospitalized children, and are positioned well to address the interests and needs of community and urban, teaching and non-teaching facilities, and the children and families they serve. These competencies reflect the areas of focused practice which, similar to pediatric emergency medicine, will no doubt be refined but not fundamentally changed in future years. The intent, we hope, is clear: to provide excellence in clinical care, accountability for practice, and lead improvements in healthcare for hospitalized children.

Address for correspondence and reprint requests:
Erin R. Stucky, MD, FAAP, FHM, 3020 Children's Way MC 5064, San Diego, CA 92123; Tel: (858)966-5841; Fax: (858) 966-6728; E-mail: estucky@rchsd.org
Received 19 January 2010; revision received 26 March 2010; accepted 26 March 2010

REFERENCES

1. Society of Hospital Medicine (SHM). Definition of a Hospitalist. http://www.hospitalmedicine.org/AM/Template.cfm?Section=General_Information&Template=/CM/HTMLDisplay.cfm&ContentID=14048. Published 2009. Accessed January 6, 2010.
2. Niccole Alexander MPP Manager Division of Hospital and Surgical Services. Pediatric Hospitalist Membership Numbers. In. Elk Grove: American Academy of Pediatrics (AAP) Section on Hospital Medicine, 141 Northwest Point Boulevard, Elk Grove Village, IL 60007; 2009.
3. Todd von Deak MBA CAE Vice President Membership and Marketing. Pediatric Hospitalists Membership Numbers. In. Philadelphia: Society of Hospital Medicine National Office 1500 Spring Garden, Suite 501, Philadelphia, PA 19130; 2009.
4. Wachter RM, L G. The emerging role of "hospitalists" in the American health care system. *N Engl J Med*. 1996;335:514–517.
5. Williams MV. The future of hospital medicine: evolution or revolution? *Am J Med*. 2004;117:446–450.
6. Wachter RM, L G. The hospitalist movement 5 years later. *JAMA*. 2002; 287:487–494.
7. Landrigan CP, Conway PH, Stucky ER, Chiang VW, Ottolini MC. Variation in pediatric hospitalists' use of proven and unproven therapies: A study from the Pediatric Research in Inpatient Settings (PRIS) network. *Journal of Hospital Medicine*. 2008;3(4):292–298.
8. Freed GL, Dunham KM, Pediatrics RACotABo. Pediatric hospitalists: Training, current practice, and career goals. *Journal of Hospital Medicine*. 2009;4(3):179–186.
9. Kurtin P, Stucky E. Standardize to Excellence: Improving the Quality and Safety of Care with Clinical Pathways. *Pediatric Clinics of North America*. 2009;56(4):893–904.
10. Stucky ER. Evolution of a new specialty - a twenty year pediatric hospitalist experience [Abstract]. In: National Association of Inpatient Physicians (now Society of Hospital Medicine). New Orleans, Louisiana; 1999.
11. Lye PS, Rauch DA, Ottolini MC, Landrigan CP, Chiang VW, Srivastava R, et al. Pediatric Hospitalists: Report of a Leadership Conference. *Pediatrics*. 2006;117(4):1122–1130.
12. Pistoria MJ, Amin AN, Dressler DD, McKean SCW, Budnitz TL e. The Core Competencies in Hospital Medicine: A Framework for Curriculum Development. *J Hosp Med*. 2006;1(Suppl 1).
13. American Board of Internal Medicine. Questions and Answers regarding ABIM Recognition of Focused Practice in Hospital Medicine through Maintenance of Certification. http://www.abim.org/news/news/focused-practice-hospital-medicine-qa.aspx. Published 2010. Accessed January 6, 2010.
14. Ingelfinger JR. Comprehensive Pediatric Hospital Medicine. *N Engl J Med*. 2008;358(21):2301–2302.
15. The Joint Commission. Performance Measurement Initiatives. http://www.jointcommission.org/PerformanceMeasurement/PerformanceMeasurement/. Published 2010. Accessed December 5, 2010.
16. The Joint Commission. Standards Frequently Asked Questions: Comprehensive Accreditation Manual for Critical Access Hospitals (CAMCAH). http://www.jointcommission.org/AccreditationPrograms/CriticalAccess Hospitals/Standards/09_FAQs/default.htm. Accessed December 5, 2008; December 14, 2009.
17. Yorita KL, Holman RC, Sejvar JJ, Steiner CA, Schonberger LB. Infectious Disease Hospitalizations Among Infants in the United States. *Pediatrics*. 2008;121(2):244–252.
18. Elixhauser A, Klemstine K, Steiner C, Bierman A. Procedures in U.S. Hospitals, 1997. HCUP Fact Book No. 2. In: Agency for Healthcare Research and Quality, Rockville, MD; 2001.
19. Anderson L, Krathwohl DR, Airasian PW, Cruikshank KA, Mayer RE, Pintrich PR, et al., editors. A Taxonomy for Learning, Teaching, and Assessing — A Revision of Bloom's Taxonomy of Educational Objectives. Addison Wesley Longman, Inc. Pearson Education USA, One Lake Street Upper Saddle River, NJ; (2001).

2010 Society of Hospital Medicine DOI 10.1002/jhm.774

Published online in wiley InterScience (www.interscience.wiley.com).